PHENOMENAL CONSCIOUSNESS

T0325310

PHENOMENAL CONSCIOUSNESS

Understanding the Relation between
Experience and Neural Processes in the Brain

Dimitris Platchias

McGill-Queen's University Press
Montreal & Kingston • Ithaca

To Maria

© Dimitris Platchias 2011

ISBN 978-0-7735-3834-4 (cloth)
ISBN 978-0-7735-3835-1 (paper)

Legal deposit first quarter 2011
Bibliothèque nationale du Québec

Published simultaneously outside North America
by Acumen Publishing Limited

McGill-Queen's University Press acknowledges the financial support of the
Government of Canada through the Canada Book Fund for its activities.

Library and Archives Canada Cataloguing in Publication

Platchias, Dimitris, 1977-
    Phenomenal consciousness : understanding the relation between
experience and neural processes in the brain / Dimitris Platchias.

Includes bibliographical references and index.
ISBN 978-0-7735-3834-4 (bound).--ISBN 978-0-7735-3835-1 (pbk.)

    1. Consciousness. 2. Experience. 3. Brain. 4. Philosophy of mind.
I. Title.

BD418.3.P63 2010   128.2   C2010-906331-7

Printed in the UK by MPG Books Group.

CONTENTS

ACKNOWLEDGEMENTS

The relation between the diverse experiences that we associate with consciousness and physical properties and how the former fit into our conception of the world has been proved very difficult and it is the central issue in the philosophy of mind. This book offers an overview of this hotly debated and rapidly developing topic – to a large extent owing to recent empirical developments – by focusing on the important philosophical and scientific work that has been done over the past thirty years in consciousness studies. This introductory approach is combined with an actual engagement in the debate and with an attempt to develop and defend a particular position.

The book has been developed on the basis of my teaching at the Departments of Philosophy of the Universities of Glasgow and Essex. The comments of my students have been invaluable and I wish to use this opportunity to thank them for their contribution. I also owe tremendous thanks to my teachers who led me to think about the way I should go about doing philosophy: Jim Edwards and Gary Kemp. Their philosophical insight and advice had a large influence on this work and made it far better than it could have been otherwise.

I have also benefited greatly from conversations with my colleagues at Glasgow and Essex, especially Fiona Macpherson, David Bain, Michael Brady and Philip Percival (Glasgow) and David McNeill, Dan Watts and Béatrice Han-Pile (Essex). I should also like to thank Scott Sturgeon and Tim Crane for their philosophical comments and our discussions. Last, but not least, thanks to two anonymous referees for their helpful comments and to my editor Tristan Palmer at Acumen for the support and the helpful manner of his collaboration.

The masters say that there is one power, by which the eye sees, and another power, by which it knows that it sees.

Meister Eckhart, *The Nobleman*

INTRODUCTION

Philosophers of mind are frequently faced with the following question: if you are interested in the mind, why not study brain science or psychology or artificial intelligence as opposed to philosophy? Another question often asked is: how can philosophy possibly contribute to our understanding of the workings of the brain and the nature of cognition and perception in general; or how can it possibly add anything to the ever-increasing wealth of empirical findings brought to light by cognitive scientists and neuroscientists in recent years? Philosophers generally respond that philosophy is (partly) concerned to find out which sciences are relevant and in what way they are relevant. However, this may not seem satisfying enough since what the above questions really amount to is: why should the study of the mind be a topic for philosophy *at all* as opposed to the sciences?

Well, in doing philosophy we can study the sort of answer that *is* required and then leave science to fill in the empirical details. And the truth is that the question of how we come to know about the nature of the mind is particularly difficult and vexing. Take, for instance, the common-sense view about people's *mental* states, such as beliefs, emotions and perceptual experiences. The general – intuitive – idea seems to be (even among scientists) that people's mental states are *essentially private* and *inaccessible* from a third-person perspective. There is some sort of access, a certain *type* of access we seem to have to our mental states, such that a mental state such as a toothache, or an emotional feeling such as being in love, is enjoyed by a *single* subject: the person who finds himself or herself in that mental state.

Ask yourself the question: can your dentist, literally speaking, see, touch or hear your toothache? You might try to describe it to your dentist, or complain about it, and your dentist may then go about discovering that you have a decayed tooth with an exposed pulp. However, it seems that your dentist cannot really perceive nor have any access to your toothache by means of any of her five modalities: the feeling of pain is just for you – no one else can have it. It seems that *you* can only have access to it by introspection or by reflecting on it and only *you* can really know what your toothache experience is like. Similarly with your emotional feeling: your best friend may notice a change in your behaviour, say absentmindedness or the speed of your reactions, and she might even be tempted to measure your blood pressure. Still, she will not be able to have any access to the feeling of love itself: the feeling of being in love is just for you – no one else can have it. It seems that it is nowhere to be seen or touched or heard, yet it somehow exists. This line of argument suggests that only you can really know in *what* kind of mental state you find yourself and only you can really know *that* you find yourself in that state. In other words, it seems that only you can really know that you have a mind.

This contrasts sharply with the knowledge or access we have of – unproblematically *physical* – tables, chairs, cars and people's bodies. There is no similar privacy there. Although there is a sense of ownership in play, physical objects are intersubjectively accessible and available for inspection. Further, physical objects frequently change hands: I can donate my car to a charity if I want to, be an organ donor or donate my body to science. No problem. No similar worries are raised here. Is this picture correct? Well, if it is then, given that the standard explanations in science are cast in objective terms (they are descriptive, they are given from a third-person perspective) and minds are subjective, it appears that minds and their mental states are not subject to the standard methods of science; they are *un*amenable to – direct – scientific investigation. This would mean that minds are not the sort of thing that can be studied by doing science. But even if this picture is not correct, its existence raises a deep philosophical question: is the mind susceptible to scientific investigation?

The problem of the relation between the various experiences that we associate with consciousness and physical properties and how it fits into our conception of the world has proved very difficult. Arguably, consciousness did not come to the higher animals as a sudden illumination. As with life originating in the pre-biotic world, consciousness came secretly and surreptitiously into a hitherto mindless world. Mammals have a cerebral cortex qualitatively similar to ours. It has been argued that consciousness occurred initially in the primitive cerebral cortices of evolving mammals such as the basal insectivores of today. It appears that consciousness is built on the anatomical and functional properties of the mammalian neocortex. However, unlike the case of life, consciousness poses a great mystery. There are a number of purported answers to the question of how physical systems that can be exhaustively explained objectively in terms of function and structure can give rise to consciousness, but none of them appears to be satisfactory. In the case of life, we had to appeal to the biological level for an explanation.

Unlike the case of consciousness, life was eventually reduced to a number of such biological functions as reproduction, development, growth, metabolism, self-repair and immunological self-defence. However, in the past thirty years, with renewed interest in studies of consciousness and the revival of neo-Cartesianism, consciousness has acquired the status of a real mystery.

Contemporary neuroscience is teaching us that our mental states correlate with neural processes in the brain. However, although we know that consciousness arises from a physical basis, we do not currently have a good explanation of *why* and *how* it so arises. Pain experiences for instance, correlate with C-fibre stimulation in the brain, but even if we know that the feeling of pain correlates with C-fibre stimulation and that, say, the existence of such pain states depends on the occurrence of such neural events (i.e. the feeling of pain is a product of the brain), we still want to know why it does not correlate with a neural state of another kind or why it is pain rather than the feeling of elation or an itch that correlates with that particular kind of neural state. This leads us to the more general question of why is it that there holds such a correlation *at all*. Trying to answer such questions raises the problem of the explanatory gap.

The explanatory gap problem has emerged into prominence in the second half of the twentieth century owing to the developed scientific worldview and the difficulty of fitting consciousness into the scientific domain, but the underlying idea, namely that human experience or consciousness cannot be fully explained by mechanical processes, is not new. Some 350 years ago, for instance, John Locke claimed in A*n Essay Concerning Human Understanding* that there is no similitude, that is similarity, between the ideas of secondary qualities (e.g. red or blue sense impressions) and the insensible particles of matter that in different degrees and modifications of their motions cause these ideas. According to him, it is not impossible to conceive then that "God should annex such ideas to such motions and that he should also annex the idea of pain to the motion of a piece of steel dividing our flesh, with which that idea has no resemblance" (1989: bk II, ch. VIII, §13).

Around the same time, Gottfried Leibniz wrote about the supposed "Mill of Perception" in his *Monadology* that:

> one is obliged to admit that *perception* and what depends upon it is *inexplicable on mechanical principles*, that is, by figures and motions. In imagining that there were a machine whose construction would enable it to think, to sense, and to have perception, one could conceive it enlarged while retaining the same proportions, so that we could enter into it, just like into a windmill. Supposing this, one should, when visiting within it, find only part pushing one another, and never anything to explain a perception. Therefore

> it is in the simple substance, and not in the composite or in the
> machine that one must look for perception.
>
> (1965: 17, emphasis added)

Why is it that certain neurophysiological processes in the brain are accompanied by *experience*? How can the richness of our mental lives arise from, as Vilayanur Ramachandran puts it, "the flux of ions in little bits of jelly – the neurons – in the brain" (2003: 112)? As Thomas Huxley once put it, this seems "just as unaccountable as the appearance of the Djinn when Aladdin rubbed his lamp" (1900: 210). This problem of *how* physical processes can give rise to experience is currently referred to as the "hard problem" of consciousness (after Chalmers 1996). To be sure, there are other problems in consciousness studies besides the hard problem, and none of them is easy. There is, for example, the problem of what we are conscious *of* or *where* in the brain consciousness arises. However interesting these questions and useful their corresponding findings may be, most philosophers currently agree that they do not give any insight into *what* explains the occurrence of our *subjective feels*; namely, to *why* physical states are accompanied by experience at all. How can the fine-grained phenomenology of conscious experience arise from neural processes in the brain? How does a set of action potentials (nerve impulses) become like the feeling of pain in one's experience?

Responses to this challenge vary widely. David Chalmers (1996) himself, for instance, thinks that the hard problem lies outside the domain of science. He thinks no explanation is possible unless we add *proto-consciousness* to our basic inventory of natural categories: a proposal not very different from what our proto-explanatory gapists above have suggested. Colin McGinn (2004) proposes that human beings are cognitively closed with respect to the solution to the problem. According to the so-called "mysterian", the explanation of the hard problem is beyond our powers of understanding; just as our ancestor *Homo habilis* cannot understand the truths of quantum physics or solve mathematical problems, we cannot solve the hard problem.[1] On the other hand, as it were, there are philosophers who take the opposite view. According to them, the explanatory reduction of consciousness in naturalistic terms *is* tractable (e.g. Block & Stalnaker 1999; Tye 2000; Rosenthal 2006). Finally, there are philosophers who think that the hard problem of consciousness is a fiction of bad philosophy and, as such, need be not explained, but explained away (e.g. Patricia Churchland 1983, and possibly Dennett 1991a).

In addition, there are now a large number of empirical findings brought to light by cognitive scientists and neuroscientists, such as the phenomenon of blindsight, change blindness, visual-form agnosia and optic ataxia, mirror recognition in other primates and split-brain cases (to mention but a few). The recently uncovered phenomena in the brain and behaviour are immensely relevant to the nature of the explanatory gap problem (or the hard problem of consciousness). It is our task to determine the extent to which these phenomena confirm or confute philosophical accounts of perception and consciousness or suggest new philosophical approaches. Furthermore, there are now a number of criticisms and recent developments in some of the most popular naturalistic theories of consciousness of the past couple of decades, such as representationalism, that need extensive treatment.

In this book, I aim to explain the key concepts that surround the hard problem of consciousness and to articulate and assess several important approaches to it, thereby giving a comprehensive treatment of the phenomenon in light of recent developments in the field. I aim to give the reader something definite and stimulating to think about, rather than to present a careful and disinterested survey of the state of the subject. In addition, and throughout the book (except Chapter 1) I attempt to defend a particular position: I formulate a higher-order thought theory of consciousness and I argue that taking consciousness to essentially involve such higher-order thought, when suitably developed, renders the explanatory reduction of consciousness in naturalistic terms tractable.

The structure of this book is as follows. In Chapter 1, I survey the main philosophical positions on the nature of mentality, thus locating the subject matter of the book within broader discussions of the mind–body problem. In Chapter 2, I explain the notion of "phenomenal consciousness", thereby disentangling it from other commonly used concepts of consciousness and I show more exactly why phenomenal consciousness is held to be the "hard" problem of consciousness as opposed to the "easy" problems. In addition, I clear up the relation between the notions of "phenomenal consciousness", "experience" and "qualia" that have been the source of so much controversy in contemporary philosophy of mind.

Next (Chapter 3), I consider the commonly held assumption that the qualitative properties of our sensory experiences, such as a pain or an itch in one's finger, are essentially conscious. That is, if one is in a mental state with one of these properties then one is in a conscious state. According to most philosophers, although many types of mental states such as thoughts, desires and beliefs can occur unconsciously – and hence "mentality" is not synonymous with "consciousness" – our qualitative states or properties are nevertheless essentially conscious, involving a different kind of consciousness: "phenomenal consciousness". In other words, some philosophers seem to think that mental qualitative properties somehow carry a (unique) kind of consciousness within themselves. If that is so, that is, if "seeing something bluish" and "seeing something yellowish", for instance, are essentially conscious, then consciousness is unanalysable and it is very unlikely that we could get any informative explanation of what being conscious consists in. However, by appealing to recent neuroscientific findings and to some philosophical thought experiments, I argue that we have no reason to hold on to this long-standing tradition. To this effect, I present and assess the Chalmers–Block view, for two reasons. First, it provides an exemplary case of a well-worked and highly influential variant of the idea that our sensory and perceptual states are essentially conscious and, second, it exemplifies that this assumption is consistent with a wide range of positions in the subject in that Chalmers is a non-reductive functionalist (ontological dualist) and Ned Block is an anti-functionalist reductionist (not a dualist).

In Chapter 4, I present and discuss Franz Brentano's notion of intentionality and consider whether phenomenal consciousness can be understood in intentional or representational terms. I consider phenomenal externalism, currently one of the most popular naturalistic approaches, and discuss in detail the main argument for the view, that is, the argument from transparency of experience. In addition, I look into Michael Tye's and Fred Dretske's neo-Brentanian naturalist versions of intentionalism and show that they do not hold what they promise. In effect, I argue that all versions of first-order (dispositionalist) intentionalism (including Daniel Dennett's) fall short of accounting for the relevant phenomena. I conclude that a theory of what it is to be conscious *of* should be kept distinct from a theory of what the objects of this consciousness are.

In Chapter 5, I specify the problem of the explanatory gap more exactly and present the kind of explanation that is required to close it. It will become clear that this neo-Cartesian challenge is indeed a very serious challenge to all physicalist and non-physicalist accounts of consciousness. I consider the main approaches to the problem (including brain-identity theory, panpsychism, McGinn's mysterianism and John Searle's biological emergentism), and becomes apparent that we are left with an unbridgeable – at least in the foreseeable future – explanatory gap: an appeal to neuroscience is the wrong level of explanation, and non-reductive and non-physicalist accounts fall short of providing the required explanation. But there is an alternative. I suggest that we should look for an explanation at the cognitive level.

In Chapter 6, I look at the main higher-order intentionalist (or representationalist) approaches. It is generally a central commitment of such theories of consciousness that they provide a reductive account of consciousness. But how exactly such theories are reductive has not been explored in much detail. In this chapter, I formulate a reductivist higher-order thought theory of consciousness and show how we can employ this theory in order to solve the problem of the explanatory gap. I conclude by addressing some of the standard objections to higher-order thought theories of consciousness, including the recently emerged and widely accepted idea that the content of our perceptual experiences is non-conceptual.

1. THE NATURE OF THE MIND

1.1 SUBSTANCE DUALISM

In this chapter, I shall present the main philosophical positions on the nature of mentality, such as substance dualism, physicalism and functionalism. This will enable us to locate the subject matter of this book within broader discussions of the mind–body problem. In this section, I shall look at substance dualism and, in particular, at the Cartesian conception of the mind. René Descartes' project in the *Meditations on First Philosophy* is a quest for indubitable truths. Descartes famously applies the method of universal doubt to "all things" in an attempt to empty the mind completely of all traditional views and preconceived ideas in order to show beyond all further doubt that truth is possible. To do this, he lays down three increasingly powerful layers of doubt. He begins his enquiry by doubting the "deliverances" or the "testimony" of the senses. Surely there is a clear sense in which our senses can deceive us; cases of perceptual error, such as illusions and hallucination, are suggestive enough. His next step was to claim that he sees "so manifestly that there are no certain indications by which we may clearly distinguish wakefulness from sleep that I am lost in astonishment. And my astonishment is such that it is almost capable of persuading me that I now dream" (1996: 13). According to Descartes, since his vivid dreams were indistinguishable from waking experience, it was possible that everything he "saw" to be part of the external (physical) world outside him was, in fact, nothing more than a fabrication of his own imagination. It was then possible to doubt that any physical thing really existed or whether there was an external world at all. Descartes' final step was to introduce the "demon" hypothesis: the possibility that there is "a malignant demon who is at once exceedingly potent and deceitful" (1998: 12) that not even these items of knowledge can survive.

These three grounds of doubt share the same structure: the senses may or may not deceive you, you may or may not be dreaming, and there may or may not be a demon around trying to deceive you at all times. The underlying idea is that we think we are in the *good* circumstance where our experiences are veridical and accurate, or where we are not dreaming and an external world exists, or where there is no deceitful demon. However, we might be in the *bad* circumstance where the opposite is true and where an evil demon is deceiving us. Our evidence would be just the same in the bad circumstance as in the good circumstance. Therefore we cannot know that we are in the good circumstance rather than in the bad: since our evidence in the good circumstance is the same as in the bad circumstance (there are no distinguishing marks between them) then even if we are in the good circumstance, we do not know that we are.

Descartes eventually lands on a bedrock certainty capable of withstanding even his worries about a deceptive demon: "But I have convinced myself that there is absolutely nothing in the world, no sky, no earth, no minds, no bodies. Does it follow from that I too do not exist? No: if I convinced myself of something then I certainly existed" (1996: 16–17). If I can be deceived, then I must exist. *Cogito ergo sum.* From establishing *that I am*, Descartes wants to know *what I am.* Following his general line of argument, it seems that one cannot say more than "I am a thing that thinks", *res cogitans.* Thinking that one has a body, or big arms, or that, say, he was born in Greece, are all immediately vulnerable to doubt. All that Descartes seems to know as to his nature is that he is a thinking thing, not that, say, he has a body. He can doubt that he has a body, but he cannot doubt that he has a mind.[1]

This can be summarized in what some philosophers call the *Cartesian epistemological argument* for the idea that minds and bodies are distinct, as follows:

> P1. I cannot doubt that my mind exists.
> P2. I can doubt that my body exists.
> Conclusion. My mind is not identical with my body.

How good is this argument? Arguments are generally tested for validity and soundness. An argument is *valid* if it is impossible for its premises to be true and its conclusion false. Here is an example:

> P1. Andrea Bocelli is an opera singer.
> P2. All opera singers are musicians.
> Conclusion. Andrea Bocelli is a musician.

When we ask whether an argument is valid or invalid we look at the argument as a whole to see whether its premises are related in this particular way: it would be impossible for the premises to be true but the conclusion false.

If an argument is invalid then even if the premises were true, it would still be possible for the conclusion to be false. In other words, if the argument is invalid then the conclusion does not follow from the premises. An argument is *sound* if and only if it is valid and all its premises are (actually) true. So if the argument is valid, this means that *if* the premises are true then the conclusion cannot be false. Hence, if the argument is valid, it is worthwhile examining whether the premises are in fact true. Since a sound argument is a valid argument with true premises, it follows that there cannot be a sound argument with a false conclusion. There are, then, two steps in assessing an argument (in that order): test the argument for validity and test the argument for soundness.

So, is the above stated argument valid? This argument has the following structure:

> P1. I cannot doubt that a is F.
> P2. I can doubt that b is F
> Conclusion. $a \neq b$

If we can find an argument with this form, then, that has true premises and a false conclusion, we will know that this argument is not valid.

> P1. I cannot doubt that Spiderman is Spiderman.
> P2. I can doubt that Peter Parker is Spiderman.
> Conclusion. Spiderman $\neq$ Peter Parker.

You can imagine a situation where both P1 and P2 are true (e.g. Gwen Stacy, Peter's first girlfriend, was in this situation) but obviously the conclusion is false. So even if both premises of the epistemological argument were true, that would not be sufficient for establishing the truth of the conclusion. Here is another example where both premises are true but the conclusion is false:

> P1. I cannot doubt that 12 is 12.
> P2. I can doubt that $\sqrt[3]{1728}$ is 12.
> Conclusion. $12 \neq \sqrt[3]{1728}$.

So the epistemological argument is not valid and we should not believe that the mind is not the body because of it.[2]

Descartes however, observes a number of differences between minds and bodies. According to him, there are certain attributes that can be ascribed to minds only and not to bodies, and vice versa. If that is right, then it does make sense to say that the mind is not the same thing as the body. This is because of Leibniz's *law of the indiscernibility of identicals*, crudely put as follows: X is the same thing as Y if and only if (iff) whatever is true of X is also true of Y or, in other words, iff whatever holds for X holds also for Y.[3]

Recall the Spiderman example. Although it does not make much sense to ask if Peter Parker is Peter Parker (or if Spiderman is Spiderman, for that matter), it makes perfect sense to ask if Peter Parker is the same person as Spiderman. Are they the same person? If they are, then it must be the case that whatever is true of Peter Parker it is also true of Spiderman. It cannot be for instance, that Peter Parker occupies a certain location in space at a certain time and Spiderman is not there, or that Spiderman is to the left or to the right of Peter Parker (as it happens with things that are qualitatively, but not numerically identical, such as identical twins or MP3 players).

The apparent differences between minds and the bodies – that certain things are true of only the former and certain other things are true of only the latter – led Descartes to the conclusion that minds and bodies are, in fact, distinct. But he did not stop there. Descartes observed that the differences between minds and bodies were so eminent and of such a fundamental nature that he exclaimed that minds and bodies are not only distinct or different things, but that they are different *kinds* of things; they are different *substances*, made of *fundamentally* different *stuff*, mental and material (or physical) stuff, respectively. In his view, a human person is a composite entity consisting of a mind and a body, each of which is an entity in its own right.

According to Descartes, then, in a position invariably called *substance dualism*, there are two sorts of substance: mental and material (or physical). These are substances of two fundamentally and irreducibly distinct kinds in this world; namely, minds and bodies. A "substance", according to Descartes, is a thing that exists in such a way as to stand in need of nothing beyond itself in order to exist. The main characteristic of a substance is the capacity for independent existence. So if you think that minds and bodies are different substances then they need nothing beyond themselves in order to exist, that is, they do not depend on each other in order to exist: the mind can exist without the body existing and vice versa.[4]

A helpful way to imagine a "substance" is to think of it as some sort of an object that persists through time. Objects (or things) are subjects of predication, that is, we normally attribute predicates or properties to them, such as "green", "tall", "low-fat", "fast" or "to the left of". Objects do not have to be concrete; we attribute properties to human and non-human primates and to chairs and tables but we also attribute properties to things such as clouds, flames and the sea. But we cannot attribute them, both concrete and non-concrete objects, to anything else. Further, the properties attributed to those objects cannot exist without these objects existing: "redness" cannot exist without the rose existing and "small" and "cuteness" cannot exist without the piggybank existing. A substance, then, can be thought of as an object that persists through time and changes, and has properties the existence of which requires the existence of the object.[5]

In what respects, then, do minds and bodies differ according to Descartes? As I said in the Introduction, it seems plausible to say that bodies can be accessed by means of the five senses and our knowledge of them involves precisely the exercise of our five modalities (and, possibly, proprioception). Contrariwise, knowledge of minds seems to necessarily involve the exercise of introspection, that is, the capacity to reflect on our mental lives, not perception. Thus, no matter how accurate your brain scanning is, no matter whether you are using positron emission tomography (PET) or functional magnetic resonance imaging (fMRI) scanning, or even if you use a very advanced technique and painlessly cut someone's brain open, you will not be able to spot any of their perceptual experiences, beliefs or desires. Further, it seems that bodies, and material objects in general, have a location in space as well as properties, such as shape, size, weight and spatial orientation, whereas minds do not; you do not find yourself saying things such as "there's a mind over there", or "my beliefs are behind or to the left of this chair", or "my memories of 2009 are 9 feet long and weight 14 stones". Mental states just do not seem to be the sorts of things that are here or there or anywhere in the relevant sense and do not have any of the above characteristics that we normally attribute to material objects, or so it seems. Finally, it seems that minds can think and understand and imagine whereas bodies do not: intuitively, you do not believe that your body or your brain cells can, strictly speaking, understand, nor do you think that when John Lennon asks you to "imagine all the people living life in peace" he invites your left arm or medial temporal lobe of your brain to do this (Table 1.1).

There are other variants of substance dualism, apart from Descartes', such as Leibniz's parallelism, Malebranche's occasionalism and Huxley's epiphenomenalism. The main difference between these views and Cartesian dualism is that Descartes held that the mind and the body could causally interact: *minds and bodies causally influence each other; some mental phenomena are*

Table 1.1 Summary of the differences between mental and material substance according to Descartes.

Physical substance: *res extensa*	Mental substance: *res cogitans*
Extended in space	Not extended in space
Has a spatial location	Has no spatial location
Not a thinking thing	Of essence a thinking thing
Known by perception	Known by introspection

causes of physical phenomena and vice versa. This view is called *interaction-ist dualism.* Indeed, if you hold a substance dualist position, *interactionism* would seem the obvious position for there seem to be obvious truths of the following kind:

Physical → causes → mental

Light hitting your eyes will *cause* you to have a visual experience.

Mental → causes → physical

Your decision can *cause* your arm to move.

If you are not careful enough and touch the red-hot oven with bare hands, then this will most probably *cause* pain in your finger, which, in turn, will *cause* a rapid withdrawal of your hand. It is certainly most natural to think that the *direct* cause of the hand withdrawal is the feeling of pain itself.[6]

All that said, in the remainder of this section, I shall be examining two arguments for substance dualism and I shall then look at some problems for the view, including mental causation problems. The first of these arguments, what might be called the Leibnizian version of the *Cartesian empirical argument* for dualism, might be stated as follows:

P1. Minds can think, understand, imagine and so on. Mere physical things (bodies) cannot.

P2. Mere physical things (bodies) are extended in space and are divisible. Minds are not divisible and do not have extension.

P3. By Leibniz law of identity: x is the same thing as y iff whatever is true of x is also true of y (or whatever holds for x holds also for y).

Conclusion. Therefore, minds and bodies are distinct.

The argument is valid, but is it sound? Granted that P3 is true, we can ask: are P1 and P2 true? Notice that this argument does not require the truth of both P1 and P2. Truth of at least one of these premises suffices. If there is at least one thing that is true of only minds and not bodies, or vice versa, then by Leibniz's law of identity minds and bodies are distinct. So if one is not tempted by dualism and wishes to reject this argument then one should pro-vide reasons to the effect that both P1 and P2 are false.

Let us start with P2. The thought that bodies are divisible and minds are not has some intuitive appeal. How could you possibly divide a mind or split it into two? However, *split-brain* cases suggest that minds, too, are divisible. It has recently been discovered that under experimental conditions, the two brain hemispheres *could* simultaneously maintain very different interpretations of the same stimulus. Our two brain hemispheres are specialized: the left hemisphere for language and speech and major problem-solving capacities and the right hemisphere for tasks such as facial recognition and attentional monitoring. In a normal brain, stimuli entering one hemisphere is quickly communicated by way of the *corpus callosum* to the other hemisphere, so the brain functions as a unit. In split-brain cases, the corpus callosum connecting the two hemispheres of the brain is severed to some degree, either as a result of an accidental injury, or by surgical operation called corpus callosotomy.[7]

When the left and right hemispheres are unable to communicate with each other, visual information no longer moves between the two sides. Michael Gazzaniga writes:

> If an image was projected to the right visual field – that is, to the left hemisphere, which is where information from the right field is processed – the patients could describe what they saw. But when the same image was displayed to the left visual field, the patients drew a blank: they said they didn't see anything. Yet if the patients were asked to point to an object similar to the one being projected, they could do so with ease. The right brain saw the image and could mobilize a nonverbal response. It simply couldn't talk about what it saw.
> (1998: 51)

Psychologist Rita Atkinson writes about Paul's case:

> It started when Paul awoke from surgery. He was immediately able to understand many kinds of language ... Instead of wondering whether or not Paul's right hemisphere was sufficiently powerful to be dubbed conscious, we were now in a position to ask Paul's right side about its views on matters of friendship, love, hate, and aspirations. "Who are you?" He writes: "Paul." "Where are you?" He writes: "Vermont." "What do you want to be?" He writes: "Automobile racer." When the left hemisphere was asked this same question, he wrote (with his right hand), "Draftsman".
> (1993: 36)

More startlingly, Ramachandran, one of the main figures in La Jolla's "neuron valley" in San Diego, discusses in the Reith Lectures a number of ways that neuroscientists today can test the personality and aesthetic preferences of the two hemispheres and describes a similar case:

13

> Imagine our surprise when we noticed that in patient LB the left hemisphere said it believed in God whereas the right hemisphere signalled that it was an atheist. The inter-trial consistency of this needs to be verified but the very least it shows that *the two hemispheres can simultaneously hold contradictory views on God.*
>
> (2003: 179, emphasis added)[8]

Notice that the relevant questions here are of considerable value to individuals. They are about the sorts of beliefs that tell us something about who we are and what we strive to be. They tell us something about our worldview and where we fit in it. Arguably, these beliefs do not and cannot exist in isolation, having nothing to do with the rest of mental life. There must be reasons for holding these beliefs. The reasons might not be good ones, but they must somehow hang together, resulting in the corresponding belief. From here, it is a short step to arrive at the idea that split-brain cases suggest that minds can be divided into two distinct articulated rationalizing structures. It seems then that minds are divisible too.[9]

What about P1? The underlying idea here is that only minds can understand and be intelligent and mere material things cannot. However, given what modern computers can do today, we might be less inclined to accept this premise. It seems that the argument begs the question, that is, it implicitly assumes what it is arguing for. Consider, on what grounds would one accept P1? Well, one of the underlying assumptions of this premise is that human beings are not "mere physical things". But if you are convinced that they are not then, in effect, you are assuming truth of the conclusion in support of P1; you are not using P1 as a reason for establishing the truth of the conclusion.[10]

Be that as it may, there is a more compelling reason to reject P1. The point succinctly put by Thomas Nagel (1986) is this, in a nutshell. If we do not understand how such states and their properties can be generated by the central nervous system, we are no closer to understanding how they might be produced by minds. So, although it might be hard to see how exactly the activity of a certain number of brain cells (or silicon chips for that matter) can constitute "understanding" or "imagining", or, to use Ramachandran's words, the activity of "the flux of ions in little bits of jelly – the neurons – in our brains" can think or understand, it is equally mysterious how minds can do these things. This point is closely related to the explanatory gap problem, about which I shall have more to say in the coming chapters. Here I merely wish to remark that the relevant question is: how can any such thing as a substance of any sort do these things? And if postulating another substance will not improve our understanding or does not create any explanatory advantage, given that this substance comes with extra explanatory burden, then we should use Ockham's razor to shave off the mental substance, because we ought not to multiply entities beyond what is necessary to explain the phenomena.

The last argument for substance dualism I shall touch on is generally called the *modal argument.* As I said above, after establishing that he exists, Descartes observes that he is essentially a *thing that thinks.* He then clearly and distinctly *conceives* of his mind existing without his body existing. This suggests to him that it is *possible* that minds and bodies are distinct and one can exist without the other. Here is the argument restated:

> P1. It is conceivable that my mind can exist without my body.
> P2. If it is conceivable that one's mind can exist without one's body then it is possible that one's mind can exist without one's body.
> Conclusion. One's mind can exist without one's body.

Of course, if the mind can exist without the body then one's mind is a different entity from one's body. Naturally, doubt here focuses on P2: why think that just because something is *conceivable* it is also a real *possibility*? There are however, problems with P1 too: can we really conceive of our mind existing without our body existing?

To be sure, imagination is a powerful tool. Think for instance, how easy it is to entertain stories such as Franz Kafka's *The Metamorphosis*, in which Gregor Samsa, a young man, transforms overnight into a giant beetle-like insect. Strictly, the only things that are unimaginable (or inconceivable) – even for a hypothetical Laplacian demon – are logical impossibilities, that is, situations where p and not-p are both true. For example, I cannot conceive of a situation where "the grass is green and the grass is not-green" or a situation where "the snow is white and the snow is not-white" (although I can conceive of a situation where "the snow is white and the snow *looks* not-white" – because say, of peculiar conditions of illumination). Now can one conceive of one's mind existing without one's body existing? Is disembodied existence conceivable?

It would initially seem that it is, but there are at least, two problems here. First, Descartes does not say much about what exactly a mental substance is. He mostly focuses on what it is not. Minds are "thinking things", which are not perceivable, not divisible and have no extension in space. This is less informative than we would hope. This line of thought led P. F. Strawson (1974) and others to argue that Cartesian dualism is not mistaken but incoherent, in the sense that there is a deep conceptual difficulty lying at the heart of the doctrine. According to Strawson, for the notion of an immaterial

Cartesian mind to make sense, it must be possible to specify criteria of *singularity* and *identity* for souls, that is, "we must know the difference between one such item and two" and "we must know how to identify the same item at different times" (*ibid.*: 173). There is no such problem with bodies: since bodies are in space as well as time we can account for their singularity and identity in spatiotemporal terms. We can appeal for instance, to a principle such as that two bodies cannot occupy exactly the same region of space at the same time. But the fact that immaterial souls are supposed to be non-spatial leaves us without any conception of what their singularity and identity consists in. Second, it might be argued that if one is convinced that minds and bodies are identical, then one cannot conceive of a situation where they are distinct; consider, is it conceivable that water and H_2O are distinct?[11]

Regarding P2, it is generally argued that although the idea that *conceivability* (or *imaginability*) implies *possibility* sounds counter-intuitive, imaginability *is* our best guide to possibility and, so far, no clear example has been produced such that one can imagine *that p* plus a good argument that it is impossible *that p*. However, it is not difficult to come up with such examples. First, we must distinguish between two notions of possibility: *nomological* and *metaphysical* possibility. Nomological possibility is possibility under the laws of nature. A certain state of affairs (*p*) is *nomologically possible* if and only if *p* is a real possibility when the physical or natural laws are as they are. On the other hand, *p* is *metaphysically possible* if and only if it is a real possibility *simpliciter*, that is, unconditionally and without any qualification. The general idea is that the laws of nature are metaphysically contingent, that is, there could have been different natural laws than the ones that actually obtain. If so, then it would not be (metaphysically) impossible, for example, that one could travel faster than the speed of light.

Let us first see why conceivability does not imply *nomological* possibility. As Gottlob Frege pointed out in his classic example, the ancients did not know that "The Morning Star" and "The Evening Star" referred to the same heavenly body, namely the planet Venus. Early astronomers could conceive, then, of the Morning Star existing without the Evening Star existing. But that was only because they were ignorant of the facts. They did not know that both descriptions referred to the same thing and therefore that was not a genuine possibility. In addition, although I *can* imagine that I could travel to Andromeda one day, that is not a real *nomological* possibility. For it would have to be the case that I could travel faster than the speed of light and so, given that the laws of nature are what they are, there is no way I could do it.

Now consider the 1985 hit film *Back to the Future*, starring Michael J. Fox. The film shows what it might be like to travel back in time, were it possible: Marty McFly winds up in a nuclear powered time-machine and is sent back in time to 1955 by his eccentric friend Dr Emmett Brown. There, he meets up with his parents to be, and realizes that his chance encounters have changed his future and therefore he must either see history repeat itself or perish. McFly's realization is important. Although it is often said that nothing can travel faster than the speed of light, there are hypothetical particles called tachyons that can travel faster that light. What the theory of relativity forbids is the transmission of *information* faster than light. The reason for this is that is easy to devise a set-up that, say, sends *signals* to the past thereby creating classic causality paradoxes.[12] So for instance, imagine that the remote control that turns the television on were able to transmit its signal into the past by two days. I could then sit the device on a radio-activated bomb, programmed to explode only if it receives a signal from the future. What will happen when I press the button after two days? The bomb would explode today, destroying the device and preventing me from pressing the button tomorrow. So although time travel is imaginable, it is deeply paradoxical and examples like this show that it is incoherent.

In addition, consider, for instance, the identification of water with H_2O. Chemistry has discovered that the liquid we call "water" is made up of molecules that are themselves made up of atoms of hydrogen and oxygen. There is nothing more to being water other than being made of H_2O. Since water and H_2O are one and the same thing, there is no situation such that one can exist without the other. In other words, it is not metaphysically possible for H_2O to exist and water not to exist. This suggests that the fact that a situation conceivable or imaginable does not mean that it is metaphysically possible. Arguably, a long time ago, natural philosophers could conceive of water existing without H_2O existing. But as it turns out that is not a genuine possibility. In a similar fashion, Nagel (1974) argues that a Presocratic philosopher could conceive that matter can exist without energy existing. But now we know that this is not a possibility. Whether we can really conceive of pains without brains, or our apparent ability to imagine one without the other, may only be due to our ignorance. It might be that identifications such as "pain = C-fibre stimulation" are necessary empirical truths, like the scientific identity "water = H_2O". Therefore, P2 is far from being true.

There are other arguments for dualism. There is, for instance, Chalmers's *conceivability argument*, often known as the *zombie hypothesis*. The argument is very similar to the Cartesian modal argument, but there are a number of important differences. Chalmers invites us to imagine the "philosophical zombie", that is, a creature that is physically, functionally and behaviourally like us. Philosophical zombies are not like Hollywood zombies; they do not move woodenly and stare fixedly. They are living organisms with which you can have a meaningful conversation. If you kick them in the knee, they will say ouch and if you scan their brains when they claim to be in pain the same bit of the brain lights up as in us non-zombies; brain processes are molecule-for-molecule identical. The zombie is practically indistinguishable from a conscious creature from a third-person point of view. But things will be different from the first-person point of view; there is nothing it is like to be them. It is all blank inside: no subjective feel accompanies their brain states. So here is the argument: since it is conceivable that all the brain states are there and mental states are not, it is possible to have the brain state without the conscious state. Since the zombie is conceivable it is – metaphysically – possible, therefore mental states are something over and above physical states.

The basic idea here is that although it does not seem possible to have H_2O without water, it does seem possible (because of the possibility of zombies) to have a brain state without a mental state; so mental states cannot be identical with any brain states. We must notice that the hypothesis is that the physical replica of the body could exist without the mind, not that the mind might continue to exist without the body, as Descartes suggests. As such, the zombie hypothesis purports to establish only property dualism, not substance dualism. For a property dualist, the mind cannot survive the death of the body. This is because on this view there is only *one* kind of substance, physical substance, having two different kinds of properties, mental and physical properties, the former not being reducible to the latter. (Recall that a substance can be thought of as an object that has properties, which cannot exist without the object existing). On this view, then, minds are not entities in their own right that can exist without bodies existing. Further, it is open for the property dualist to deny P1 of the modal argument above and hold that disembodied existence is inconceivable.[13]

There is, however, another way that the zombie hypothesis is relevant to discussions on substance dualism. This involves the idea that substance dualism is unable to account for knowledge of others' minds. The view seems to account well for our intuition that we have special access to our own minds and would explain why our minds are private. But it does not account well for the knowledge that we typically think that we have of other minds. Since dualism holds that minds are essentially private and inaccessible from a third-person point of view, it leaves open the possibility of philosophical zombies thereby making knowledge of other minds not possible at all. This flies in the face of our everyday experience, since not only do I normally think that I know that you have a mind, but I normally think that sometimes I can know *which* mental state you are in and *what* that state is like.

Furthermore, if our mental states are essentially private, how are we able to communicate them? How are we able to communicate the private contents of our inner experiences? Ludwig Wittgenstein has famously argued in the negative.[14] According to him, if we indeed had such private mental items, it would be possible to represent them in a corresponding language. The individual words of this language would refer to what can only be known to the person speaking. Call this language *private* in that the words would refer only to the person's inner *private* sensations and mental states. This means that another person cannot understand the language. But, Wittgenstein argues, such language is impossible. The very notion of such language is utterly nonsensical for Wittgenstein. The reason for this is that language has criteria of *correctness* and self-ascriptions of mental states in the present sense are not based on anything; they are, so to speak, *criterionless*. This means that when someone sincerely asserts that she possesses a sensation or that she is having a particular experience, she does not have a *reason* for believing that she does (i.e. that her sincere assertion is true). Suppose you want to keep a diary about the recurrence of a certain sensation. You associate the sensation with the sign "S" and write this sign in the calendar for every day on which you have that sensation. For this, you would have to remember the connection and write "S" in your calendar when and only when you really have S. But how can you be sure that you have remembered the sensation all right next time you call a sensation "S"? Might it not have been that you only had a very similar sensation? Further, and as opposed to everyday memory mistakes about external (public) objects, private-language mistakes cannot be corrected. There is no sort of external verification here, no set of criteria for correct application. Hence private language is impossible and, therefore, there are no such private inner experiences.

The dualist might respond that Wittgenstein's point is a point about language, that is, you cannot rule out the possibility that such private inner experiences exist simply because they cannot be represented in a corresponding language. But how are we to account for the fact that we *can* talk about our mental states and that mental expressions such as "I have a toothache" or "I have a throbbing pain in my arm" can be used to transmit information from person to person?

Wittgenstein writes:

> Suppose everyone had a box with something in it: we call it a "beetle". No one can look into anyone else's box, and everyone says he knows what a beetle is only by looking at his beetle. – Here it would be quite possible for everyone to have something different in his box. One might even imagine such a thing constantly change. – But suppose the word "beetle" had a use in these people's language – If so it would not be used as the name of a thing. The thing in the box has no place in the language-game at all; not even as a something: for the box might even be empty. – No, one can "divide through" by the thing in the box; it cancels out, whatever it is. (1953: §293)

Wittgenstein's point is that it is difficult to see how the word "beetle" can have a role in interpersonal communication. If language is to be used as means for public communication and terms such as "beetle" get their meaning only by reference to some essentially private mental sample to which only I can have access, then the mental sample ends up being irrelevant to whatever public meaning our use of the concept "beetle" might have. Thus if we can talk about something then that cannot be private in the sense that Cartesian minds are, and if it is private in that sense then we cannot talk about it. And since we can talk about our mental states, and utterances such as "I have a toothache" or "I have a throbbing pain in my arm" can be used to transmit information from person to person, expressions such as "pain" and "redness" are unlike Wittgensteinian "beetles" and they have intersubjective meanings. Hence *what* we are talking about cannot be private in the Cartesian sense. This undermines the Cartesian conception of the mind, thereby endorsing the behaviourist intuition that our mental expressions are referring to facts that are *publicly observable*, or to whatever is intersubjectively accessible and open to third-person investigation.

Cartesian interactionism faces other serious difficulties. The view seems unable to explain the possibility of mental causation, that is, the possibility that mentality makes a causal difference in the world. For, as Jaegwon Kim puts it, "it simply does not seem credible that an immaterial substance, with no material characteristics and totally outside physical space, could causally influence, and be influenced by, the motions of material bodies that are strictly governed by physical law" (2006: 4). Recall that Descartes held that mental substance is radically different from physical substance since it *does not exist in space* and *has no mass or shape*, yet minds and bodies could causally interact. But how can mental stuff interact with physical stuff when they are so different? Consider, *where* would the interaction take place? The answer is that it cannot take place *anywhere* because the mind is non-spatial; it has no location in space. However, it must take place somewhere if the physical is to be affected. In other words, for causation to take place there must be a *causal interface* located some*where*. Since there is no such interface, it is hard to see how it can take place.

There are a number of conceptual difficulties here, since, for instance, it does not make sense to say that my mind is "closer" or "nearer" to me than to you, and yet it seems that we get to hang out together all the time. And when my body leaves the room, my mind is not left *in there*. It seems that my mind is roughly (or exactly) *where* my body is, but what keeps it *there*? What keeps my mind in that particular "location"? As Kim succinctly puts it:

> the causal relation indeed exerts a strong pressure toward a degree
> of homogeneity over its domain, and, moreover, that the kind of

> homogeneity it requires includes, at a minimum, spatiotemporality, which arguably entails physicality. The more we think about causation, the clearer becomes our realisation that the possibility of causation between distinct objects depends on a shared space-like coordinate system in which these objects are located, a scheme that individuates objects by their "locations" in the scheme. Are there such schemes other than physical space? I don't believe we know of any.　　　　　　　　　　　　　　　　　　　(2005: 91)

In addition, it seems that if minds are in *time*, then they ought to be in *space* too. The concept of space–time combines space and time within a single coordinate system. Scientists talk about space–time continua as a way of describing the workings of the universe in a uniform way, both at the subatomic level and the level of clusters of galaxies. It is no longer believed, for instance, that time is independent from motion, in that several experiments have shown that the rate at which time passes depends on an object's velocity relative to the speed of light. Thus if minds are *in time* and since we generally think that mental states *are* causally efficacious, for example being in pain *causes* pain behaviour, it is very tempting to think that minds are spatiotemporal entities, that is, physical entities.

Indeed, there is a fundamental principle in physics called the *principle of the causal closure of the physical*. This involves the idea that every physical effect takes a physical cause. More precisely, according to this principle, for every physical phenomenon there is a complete causal explanation specified exclusively in physical terms. In other words, for every physical phenomenon or state there is a complete physical explanation as to *how* that phenomenon is brought about or *why* that state is realized. It might then be argued that since the physical domain is causally closed and the mind can cause physical phenomena or states, then the mind is physical too. The Cartesian interactionist claim that minds are non-physical, yet they can exert causal influence on the world, has the consequence of violating this principle.

There are three options for the substance dualist: (i) bite the very big bullet that a central principle of fundamental physics is false; (ii) appeal to overdetermination; (iii) keep "substance dualism" and change "interactionism". The first is indeed very hard to swallow. The search for physical causes of the physical has been one of the science's great success stories. Once we explained the growth of plants in terms of the vital spirit; now we explain it in terms of cell division. Once we explained thunder in terms of Zeus's anger; now we explain it in terms of the sudden increase in pressure and temperature from lightning, which produces rapid expansion of the surrounding air. Once we explained earthquakes in terms of the temperament of the giant Egelados, who was trying to struggle out from under the weight of rocks where he was put by the ancient Greek goddess Athena; now we explain them in terms of a release of energy in the earth's crust or by the movement of magma in volcanic areas.

These examples are suggestive enough. It is very hard to believe that we shall ever find evidence that when one exhibits pain behaviour, something "outside physical space" that cannot be specified in physical terms is affecting what happens. The data from neurology show that all the diverse experiences or mental phenomena correlate with particular patterns of brain activity. All we know about it with any certainty points to the fact that all these experiences are a product of brain activity and that with no brain there are no such experiences. It is hard to believe that, nevertheless, mental states are products of non-material thinking souls that exist alongside brains and somehow interact with them. Here's Descartes tale:

> Thus, for example, when the nerves in the foot are agitated in a violent and unusual manner, this motion of theirs extends through the marrow of the spine to the inner reaches of the brain, where it gives the mind the sign to sense something, namely the pain as if it is occurring in the foot … when we need something to drink, a certain dryness arises in the throat that moves the nerves in the throat, and, by means of them, the inner parts of the brain. And this motion affects the mind with a sensation of thirst.
>
> (1998: 102)

According to Descartes, as a result of the blood's functions and tendencies, animal spirits are generated "which are like a very subtle wind, or rather, like a very pure and lively flame that rises continuously in great abundance from the heart to the brain, and from there goes through the nerves into the muscles, and gives movement to all the members" (*ibid.*: 30). However, the data from neurology strongly suggest a completely different, animal-spirit-free, picture. We now know, for instance, that by inducing electrical currents in particular areas of the brain we can evoke certain – involuntary – movements, for example a joint flexes, a muscle group in the face contracts, fingers move and, in some cases, the patients adopt a certain posture, for example they extend their neck or rotate their head to the left.[15] There is a sufficient, fully satisfactory explanation as to how exactly these movements are brought about and there is no need to appeal to any sort of exotic animal spirits.

Similarly with *alien hand syndromes*. In these cases, patients typically find themselves fighting one hand with the other, or they find one hand does some activity and the other undoes it. In extreme cases, the alien hand tries to strangle the person. The patients generally report that it feels as if the hand has a mind of its own. No doubt, three hundred years ago, people would say that these people were possessed by some evil spirit or demon that makes the hand move, and that exorcism is probably the best way forwards. However, there is now a straightforward neuroscientific explanation – this condition arises from lesions in the patient's brain – and there are now a number of different strategies to reduce the inference of the alien hand behaviour on the controlled bodily actions of the patient.

Abandoning the idea that the principle of the causal closure of the physical might be false, the substance dualist might appeal to *causal overdetermination*. This is the idea that mental properties and physical properties *separately* overdetermine physical goings on in the world. Causal overdetermination means there can be two or more distinct causes of an effect, each *sufficient* by itself to bring about that effect, and both occur. So, for example, if someone is shot by two members of a firing squad, and two bullets enter the same organ at the same moment, this is a case of overdetermination in that either bullet could have done the job and both bullets hit the target. This seems to leave the principle of the causal closure unaffected in that it allows that everything in the physical world has a sufficient physical cause without excluding a causal input from mental properties. Pain behaviour in humans, then, may have two separate causes, one mental and one physical, each of which is sufficient to make this behaviour occur.

There are a number of difficulties here. First, explanations in science proceed by eliminating the relevant alternatives or the rival hypotheses. Different explanations of the same phenomenon typically exclude each other, and the exclusion of possibilities is what an informative answer consists in and what information in its broadest sense is. The explanation of thunder in terms of the increase in pressure and temperature from lightning *displaced* the explanation in terms of Zeus's anger; it was not added on. And when the electrical devices in the house stop working all at once, you normally infer that a fuse must have blown. When the blown fuse gets replaced and everything goes back to normal, the rival hypotheses are excluded, including the electricity being cut off and Zeus' anger.

Second, why postulate the existence of entities that have no work to do? An acute pain in my finger will cause me to scream ouch! Neuroscience tells us a detailed story about how exactly damaged tissue will cause a certain brain state and how this, in turn, will cause pain behaviour. The causal story is certainly much more complex than this, but the point is that if neuroscience can give us a complete causal explanation of the pain behaviour, specified exclusively in neurophysiological or physical terms, then why do we need the extra entities? Consider this. Normally, if you touch a red-hot oven with bare hands, it will cause pain in your finger, which, in turn, will cause a rapid withdrawal of your hand. The causal overdetermination story has it that there are two causes, one physical and one mental, each sufficient to bring about the effect, and that they both occur (in the brain and in the mind respectively). Now suppose that the next time you touch a hot oven, it so happens that in virtue of, say, some misfiring in the brain, the causal chain breaks down in such a way that the physical state in question does not occur; only the mental state occurs – you find yourself in pain (or suppose that although both the pain and the brain state occur, a mad scientist somehow blocks the brain state's causal potential). What would happen in this case? Will you still be withdrawing your arm? If yes, then this amounts to option (i) above: violation of causal closure. If no, then this suggests that there exists some sort of a pre-established harmony or regularity between physical and mental causes, that is, if the mental state occurs then it is sufficient to bring about a physical effect if and only if the relevant physical state also occurs and it is sufficient to bring about that effect. If so then, for one thing, one needs to explain this peculiar regularity, and, for another, it really looks like the mental has no causal work to do *at all*. Thus, since the mental entity has no explanatory or causal work to do and it comes with an extra explanatory burden, we ought to use Ockham's razor and shave it off.[16]

The third option for the substance dualist is to adopt epiphenomenalism, at the expense of abandoning causal interactionism. *Epiphenomenalism* is the view that mental phenomena are caused by physical phenomena in the brain but they do not cause any physical phenomena in turn. As the evolutionary biologist Huxley put it quite some time ago, consciousness (or all of our mental life) is like the whistle of a steam train: a by-product of the neurological complexity of the brain. This view certainly sounds deeply counter-intuitive: it seems impossible to believe that those mental states such as our thoughts and feelings have no effect on our actions and behaviour. In addition, how can we explain the evolution of consciousness if our mental life is just a side effect? Why does natural selection "prefer" or "choose" more complex states of consciousness over less complex ones if these are not to make any contribution whatever towards survival and reproduction? The standard epiphenomenalist response is that owing to psycho-physical laws (which go in only one direction, from physical to mental), the more complex the physical systems selected, the more complex the states of consciousness that evolve.

However, there are at least two problems here. First, how can we have knowledge of mental properties if they are inefficacious? For an epiphenomenalist, a mental state cannot cause the belief that one is in that state. Pain, for example, cannot cause the utterance "I'm in pain". The epiphenomenalist answer is, generally, that one and the same neural event is the cause of both the mental state and our report and it only *seems* to us that the mental state is the – direct – cause of the report. But the epiphenomenalist claim does not really square with our intuition that our perceptual experiences and bodily sensations provide *rational grounds* for the formation of our perceptual beliefs and judgements: I see that there is a cup on my desk and on that very basis I form the belief that there is cup right in front of me. My belief is neither accidental nor the result of an act of will. It is hard to see how an epiphenomenalist can account for the intuitive idea that such beliefs are the sorts of entities that can be assessed as being rational or irrational, justified or unjustified. For the epiphenomenalist treats them as brute occurrences.[17]

Second, how does the physical-to-mental direction work exactly? In other words, how do mental phenomena (being non-material or non-spatial) *arise* from material phenomena (spatial) or how could the right sort of *causation* possibly explain this? As William Robinson (2004b) observes, science explains *structure* in the causes, where the relevant structures are spatio-temporal structures, and an additional fact about structure will not seem to explain how something physical can give rise to something non-physical. In fact, that was one of the main motivations for the idea that there are two sorts of substance in this world; namely, that mental phenomena cannot be explained in terms of material or physical phenomena. What is more, epiphenomenalists accept that the physical realm is causally closed. But if so, then no brain state can *cause* a mental state for, according to the principle, as Kim puts it, "if you pick any physical event and trace out its *causal ancestry* or *posterity*, that will never take you outside the physical domain" (1998: 40). On this view then, it is hard to see how *mental* states can arise from, be determined by or be explained in terms of *physical* properties of neurons in the brain or how one can consistently maintain both that mental states are caused by the brain and that the physical is causally closed.[18]

1.2 BEHAVIOURISM

John Watson first introduced behaviourism in the early twentieth century in his paper "Psychology as the Behaviorist Views It" (1913). Watson believed that inner experiences could not be studied because they were not observable. According to him, psychology should be the science of observable behaviour: scientific theories need to be supported by empirical data obtained through careful and controlled observation and if minds are essentially private and inaccessible from a third-person point of view then they are not open to scientific investigation.

Behaviourism is primarily concerned with *observable behaviour*, as opposed to internal states of the organism, including inner mental experience and states of the brain. The latter, although they are themselves physical states, are not on the behaviourist list. By "behaviour" the behaviourist means observable (i.e. external) behaviour that can be objectively and scientifically measured (measured responses to stimuli). Generally, what is meant by "behaviour" are publicly observable and measurable conditions about people, such as bodily reactions and bodily movements, such as vocal and facial expressions, perspiration, salivation, increase in blood pressure, raising a hand, closing a window and so on. According to behaviourism, all behaviour, no matter how complex, can be reduced to a simple stimulus–response association.[19]

Behaviourism came as a reaction to the Cartesian conception of the mind. We saw previously that although substance dualism seems to account well for our intuition that we have special access to our own minds and would explain why our minds are private, it seems to make knowledge of other minds not possible at all. Wittgensteinian arguments, together with the rise of verificationism in the 1930s, discredited the Cartesian conception of the mind and suggested that we should take the meanings of mental expressions to refer to publicly accessible and intersubjectively verifiable facts about people. We saw earlier that the main idea in these arguments is that psychological expressions have shareable meanings and can be used to transmit information from person to person. Expressions such as "pain" and "redness", unlike Wittgensteinian "beetles", have intersubjective meanings. This means that statements about our mental states have meanings that are specifiable by conditions that are *publicly observable* and hence *what* we are talking *about* cannot be private in the Cartesian sense.[20]

According to behaviourism, behaviour is *constitutive* of mentality, that is to say, mentality *essentially consists in* the exhibition or the disposition to exhibit certain appropriate patterns of observable behaviour. This is not to say that there are inner mental states over and above observable behaviour that *correlate* or *cause* certain behavioural manifestations as this claim is consistent with substance dualism. The claim is rather that for a creature to have mentality *just is* for it to exhibit or have the disposition to exhibit certain appropriate patterns of behaviour. So the feeling of pain, for instance, simply *consists in* a certain appropriate behavioural pattern or a disposition to exhibit pain behaviour, such as wincing and groaning in the right environmental circumstances. All variety of mental phenomena can be defined solely in terms of observable (external) physical phenomena.[21]

The behaviourist conception of the mind is highly problematic. For one thing, some thoughts and beliefs have no behavioural realization at all (e.g. mathematical statements such as "1 + 1 = 2" or the law of non-contradiction in logic – "it cannot be the case that a proposition is both true and false"). For another, it appears that perceptual responsiveness to stimuli or exhibition of certain appropriate patterns of (observable) behaviour is neither necessary nor sufficient for, say, a pain experience. It does seem that you can feel pain without showing it and that there is a difference between being in pain and acting *as if* you are in pain. Regarding the first, it seems that lack of responsiveness or of exhibiting pain behaviour does not imply lack of pain. People with paralysed legs and hands (quadriplegics) cannot execute any movement of arms and legs, yet they feel pain and they generally find themselves in real psychological states. Relatedly, consider Hilary Putnam's "super-spartans" and "super-stoics":

> Imagine a community of "super-spartans" or "super-stoics" – a community in which the adults have the ability to successfully suppress all involuntary pain behavior. They may, on occasion, admit that they feel pain, but always in pleasant, well-modulated voices – even if they are undergoing the agonies of the damned. They do not wince, scream, flinch, sob, grit their teeth, clench their fists, exhibit beads of sweat, or otherwise act like people in pain or people suppressing the unconditioned responses associated with pain. However, they do feel pain, and they dislike it (just as we do). They even admit that it takes a great effort of will to behave as they do. It is only that they have what they regard as important ideological reasons for behaving as they do, and they have, through years of training, learned to live up to their own exacting standards.
>
> (1963: 215)

There are a number of more mundane everyday life instances, in which we find ourselves in real psychological states, but we do not alter our behaviour: people "hide" their emotions, so to speak, in order to behave in a more "emotionally intelligent" way. And there are substances, such as curare (a muscle paralysant) that can produce imprisoned minds. Curare is normally added to some anaesthetic mixes to keep surgery patients from moving. In sufficient doses, curare produces total paralysis. On regaining consciousness, the patients can feel pain but they may lose all capacity to express what they are feeling.

Conversely, lack of pain does not imply lack of responsiveness or of exhibiting certain appropriate patterns of observable behaviour. Imagine, for instance, that one is in a dreamless sleep and moves in response to a muscle cramp. This is a clear case where sensory responsiveness is not sufficient for a pain experience; there is nothing it is like for one to be in such state. Other examples may include actors, insects, robots and philosophical zombies; a creature may not find itself in genuine mental states, yet might exhibit or be disposed to exhibit the appropriate behavioural output in the right environmental circumstances.

Furthermore, according to the behaviourist, the explanation of behaviour must not involve an appeal to beliefs, desires and intentions. This is not only because the behaviourist regards such states as utterly unscientific, but also because an informative theory surely should not appeal to the very things it purports to explain (e.g. to cognitive or mental activity). However, it is hard to see how we can explain behaviour without appealing to people's beliefs and desires. The mental states people have help us explain *what* they do and *why* they do it. My *belief* that I am cold and my *desire* that I do not want to be cold coupled with my *believing* the conditional statement "if I close the window then I will not be cold", *explains* why I close the window on a cold night. Further, people are generally held accountable or morally responsible for their actions. It seems that people's behaviour is the sort of entity that can be assessed as *rational* or *irrational* and the behaviourist, by reducing all behaviour to simple stimulus–response associations, simply cannot account for this.

Finally, it is notoriously difficult to associate a unique behavioural pattern with every distinct mental phenomenon. Take the case of the emotions. It is plain that mental states such as grief and remorse have a number of different behavioural manifestations. But the same is true for less complex or cognitive emotions such as anger and fear. Anger, for instance, may involve yelling, attacking or withdrawing, and fear may involve escaping behaviour, but also attacking or freezing. In addition, and in relation to what I said in the preceding paragraph, factors other than one's immediate feeling can influence one's facial movements; for example a smile might indicate happiness, but also embarrassment or the desire to please others. Lastly, there is no distinctive bodily response corresponding to every emotion. The visceral reactions characteristic of the distinct emotions fear and anger, for instance, are identical. These reactions, then, cannot be what allow us to tell emotions apart. And imagine how difficult it would be to distinguish between very similar emotions such as guilt, embarrassment and shame by simply looking at the associated bodily reactions and/or bodily movements. These considerations suggest that we are not entitled to "read" emotions merely by observing someone's behavioural manifestations.

1.3 BRAIN-IDENTITY THEORY

According to brain-identity theory, there is nothing more to the mental than the physical states, events and processes of the brain. On a par with behaviourism, this theory is a form of reductionism because it claims that the mind is *identical* to the brain: each type of mental item is identical with some type of physical item in the brain.[22] More precisely, this view holds that for every type of mental state M, there exists a type of physical state P such that for every mental token m of type M, there exists a token physical state p of type P such that m is identical to p. So, for instance, there are several mental types, such as being in pain, being in love, being depressed and so on, and there are also different types of physical states (e.g. brain states), such as a state of certain C-fibres firing. Mental tokens are mental episodes or occurrences. So *every time* you are in pain a mental token of the type being in pain is instantiated or occurs. This view is commonly called the *type–type* identity thesis because, according to it, mental states of a certain type are identical to the physical state or process of a particular type. In other words, mental state *types* are identified with physical state *types*; for example, a mental state type, such as being in pain, is identified with a physical state type such as C-fibres firing. On this view, mental phenomena are not caused by processes or goings on in the brain; mental phenomena *just are* features of the brain.

Recall Frege's example. According to Frege, the ancients did not know that the descriptions "The Morning Star" (or "Phosphorus") and "The Evening Star" ("Hesperus") referred to the same heavenly body, Venus. So when they discovered it they learned something important: "The Morning Star is the Evening Star" ("Hesperus is Phosphorus"). This last statement is informative because "The Morning Star" and "The Evening Star" have different intensions or meanings. But they have the same extension: the thing or the set of things to which the term refer. That is, they both refer to the same object, to the same heavenly body. So when we want to speak of Venus we can use, interchangeably, both descriptions (provided, of course, that our audience are aware of both). Similarly with the statement "pain is C-fibre firing". The intension of "pain" (what the term means) is different from the intension of "C-fibre firing". Many people, for instance, know a lot about pains but nothing about C-fibre firings. Yet, on this view, the two terms pick out the same phenomenon: pain is one and the same thing as C-fibre firing. In other words, there is only one thing here, C-fibre firing (i.e. pain), which can be known under two descriptions or "modes of presentation": pain and C-fibre firing. So the statement "Pain is C-fibre firing" is, similarly, an informative identity statement.[23]

There are, in the main, two related reasons for why we should think that such mind–brain identities hold. First, contemporary neuroscience is teaching us that there are *systematic correlations* between mental phenomena and neural processes in the brain. The feeling of pain, for instance, correlates with C-fibre firing in the brain. In addition, there is overwhelming empirical evidence showing that brain lesions (sometimes intentionally inflicted during neurosurgery) may have a dramatic effect on the mental life of the individual. Further, we now know that the communication between neurons is controlled by the brain's type and level of neurotransmitters. Neurotransmitters are the chemicals that allow the transmission of signals from one neuron to the next across synapses. We have now begun to identify which neurotransmitters control certain bodily functions or which were related to certain mental conditions. A large number of studies have shown that there is a strong connection between neurotransmitters and mental conditions: the presence of specific psychiatric conditions depends and is determined by the amounts of certain neurotransmitters in the brain. This strongly suggests that there is a *relation of dependency* between mental phenomena and neural processes in the brain: Mental phenomena depend on and are determined by physical goings on in our brains. Thus, if our mental properties *systematically correlate, depend on* and are *determined by* the physical goings on in our brains, then it very much looks like that the mental is firmly anchored in the physical domain.[24]

However, even if a pain experience, for instance, correlates with C-fibre firing and the existence of such pain states is contingent on the occurrence of such a neural event we still want to know *why* it does not correlate with a neural state of another kind or why it is pain rather than the feeling of elation, say, that correlates with that particular kind of neural state. This is where the second motivation for the view kicks in: instead of trying to explain the correlation, by discovering, say, any (psycho-physical) laws that might govern the correlation, the identity theorist appeals to the principle of simplicity (Ockham's razor) and to what in science is called "inference to the best explanation", and postulates an *identity* relation: the "correlation" between, say, pain and C-fibre firing holds because in fact, they are one and the same thing. J. J. Smart writes:

> Why do I wish [to identify sensations with brain processes]? Mainly because of Occam's razor … There does seem to be, so far as science is concerned, nothing in the world but increasingly complex arrangements of physical constituents. All except for in one place: in consciousness … That these [states of consciousness] should be *correlated* with brain processes does not help, for to say they are correlated is to say that they are something "over and above" … states of consciousness seem to be the one sort of thing left outside the physicalist picture, and for various reasons I just cannot believe that this can be so. That everything be explicable.
>
> (1959: 142, emphasis added)

Indeed, the statement "*A* correlates with *B*" implies that there are two things there, or at any rate, as Smart puts it, it implies that *A* is something "over and above" *B*. For example, we do not say that water correlates with H_2O; we rather say water *is* H_2O.[25] Even if it turns out that science can establish one-to-one correlations (or correspondence, as some scientists call it) between mental and physical phenomena, the picture does not change. Suppose we discover that the same patterns of neural activity correlate with the same mental phenomena across different studies and contexts; that is, the same brain areas are implicated in the same mental phenomena and different mental phenomena do not overlap – they do not have any brain areas in common. This would reveal reliable one-to-one correlations or correspondences between individual mental phenomena and particular patterns of brain activity. But even if one establishes such correlations as "Pain occurs *if and only if* C-fibre firing occurs" (or "Pain occurs *exactly if* or *just in case* C-fibre firing occurs"), one still needs to explain these correlations. Why is it that pain correlates with C-fibre firing instead of a neural state of another kind?

One way to explain these correlations is to suggest that that there are laws that govern these correlations, thereby explaining why these correlations hold. However, the task of identifying such laws is extremely difficult, if not impossible. For what *sorts* of laws might govern, or explain the correlation between, mental and physical phenomena? Consider, why does *thunder* occur when *lightning* occurs? According to the physics of electromagnetism, there are certain *physical laws* due to which, when the difference of charge between two regions, such as that between two clouds, reaches a certain point, the air between the two regions becomes ionized (i.e. breaks down) and lightning occurs. Indeed, there are a number of physical laws that explain direct correlations between properties. The *ideal gas law,* for instance, explains the correlation between pressure and temperature: given a fixed mass, an increase in temperature will cause an increase in pressure and an increased pressure will cause an increase in temperature.

However, the laws that explain the lightning–thunder or the pressure–temperature correlation are *exclusively* physical laws, whereas the laws that would explain the pain–C-fibre firing correlation cannot be exclusively physical laws in that the concept "pain" does not feature in the physical laws; it is not part of the language of physics. So the law correlating the occurrence of pain (a psychological occurrence) and the activation of C-fibres (a neurological occurrence), that is, the law that governs the correlation between a mental and a physical phenomenon, has to be a *psycho*-physical law. But given the incredible difficulty of discovering any such laws, there is a danger that, in the end, we will simply postulate such correlations as *fundamental brute facts* about the world, that is, facts unamenable to further explanation or instigation. A very complex picture then emerges about the world: this will have to be true for every such correlation between mental phenomena and physical goings on in our brains. Together with the basic laws of nature discovered by physicists, we need to add a plethora of such psycho-physical laws to our basic inventory of fundamental natural laws.

Smart's point is that the picture is far simpler if we use Ockham's razor and shave off these laws. Consider this example again. Why does *lightning* occur whenever there is an *electrical discharge* between two clouds (or between two regions in general)? Because lightning just *is* the electrical discharge involving these regions. Similarly, why is it that pain occurs whenever C-fibre firing occurs? Because, the argument goes, they are one and the same thing: mental states or events are *identical* to neurophysiological processes in the brain.

Ontologically speaking, our explanation is now simpler in that we do not need to posit two kinds of states (mental and physical) to explain the phenomena. Further, we do not need to look for any mysterious psycho-physical laws that govern the correlation between mental states and physical states. Indeed, we saw previously that the principle of the causal closure of the physical requires a complete causal explanation of physical phenomena or events in solely physical terms. The withdrawal of your arm, after burning your hand on a hot stove, can have a complete explanation in physical terms: contemporary neuroscience can currently provide a detailed causal story from damaged tissue to pain behaviour.[26]

At the same time, we do think that that it was the pain in your finger that caused you to withdraw your arm. However, there are two ways to retain the causal efficacy of pain. We can either identify it with the physical state in your brain or appeal to causal overdetermination. Since, arguably, overdetermination is not an option, pain has to be identical with the physical state: it is either that pain is distinct from and irreducible to C-fibre firing or it is one and the same thing as C-fibre firing. If the first is true, then given that the physical is causally closed and that overdetermination is not an option, pain is an epiphenomenon; it is causally inert and it only *seems* to you that it causes your arm movement. If the second, then pain is identical to C-fibre firing in your brain and therefore it causes your arm movement. So instead of thinking of pain as being causally impotent or epiphenomenal, provided that overdetermination is not an option, we can identify it with the relevant pattern of brain activity and safeguard its causal role.[27]

Thus, it seems that the *best* way we can currently explain the correlations between mental and physical phenomena is to say that the mental phenomena are nothing over and above the physical goings on in our brains. This is immediately related to what scientists call *inference to the best explanation*, which involves the idea that where there are a number of possible hypotheses, each of which, if true, would explain the data or our observations, we should choose the *best* one. Generally, a hypothesis provides a better explanation than its competitors when it provides the *simplest* explanation, that is, the one that is conceptually and theoretically clearest, entails nothing unwanted and contains nothing unwanted. Further it must integrate and fit in well with other explanations in science, for science is a structured and coherent whole. This, in effect, results in a better understanding of mental phenomena and, in particular, of how they are related to physical phenomena. In the same way that we understand thermodynamical phenomena better when we show them to be identical with certain kinds of mechanical activity, we understand mental phenomena better when we show them to be identical with neurophysiological occurrences in the brain.

In addition, this explanation comes from a scientific discovery and coming to know that mental states are brain states via scientific investigation fleshes out the idea that only by going out into the world can we come to know that mental states are brain states. David Armstrong (1968) provides an illustrative example. Armstrong invites us to consider genes. Long before we discovered DNA, we knew about genes. Gregor Mendel, based on his work with pea plants, described how traits were inherited or passed on from parent organisms. The entity responsible for this inheritance was termed a "gene". About half a century later, Frederick Griffith was working on a project that enabled others to point out that DNA was the molecule of inheritance. Research into DNA ultimately discovered that it was portions of DNA that caused the hereditariness of certain characteristics. So an identification was made: portions of DNA = genes.

According to Armstrong, the identification was made because we defined a gene as being *that thing that played a certain causal role*. Armstrong invites us to use the same line of argument regarding mental states. Pain, for instance, seems to be some sort of an internal state that is normally caused by tissue damage and causes a certain pattern of behaviour such as wincing and groaning. Since there is overwhelming neurophysiological evidence to the effect that C-fibre firing is the internal state that is normally caused by tissue damage and that it causes a certain pattern of behaviour such as wincing and groaning, we should identify pain with C-fibre firing. As in the case of genes, we defined pain as being *the thing that plays a certain causal role* and subsequent research has uncovered what that thing is.

However, the idea that mental phenomena are identical with neurophysiological occurrences in the brain faces serious problems. I shall be briefly discussing three objections: the *knowledge argument*, Saul Kripke's *modal argument* and the *multiple realizability argument*. The knowledge argument occurs in different ways in the work of Nagel (1974) and Frank Jackson (1982) and was foreshadowed by Bertrand Russell (1918). Russell invites us to consider two propositions: a proposition *p*, which contains "the colour with the greatest wavelength", and a proposition *q*, which contains "red". Do these propositions have the same meaning? Russell says no. If you try to define "red" as "the colour with the greatest wavelength" you are not giving the meaning of the word at all. "The colour with the greatest wavelength" is simply a true description of "red"; it is not its meaning. What you mean by "red" is that *there is something it is like* for you to see that colour in immediate distinction from, say, "green" or "blue", and we cannot capture this distinction simply by appealing to wavelengths of light.

The classic statement of the knowledge argument, however, has been given by Jackson (1982). Jackson invites us to imagine Mary, a future super neuroscientist who knows all there is to know about the human brain and colour vision (even those theories that have not yet been discovered and formulated). However, she is raised in a completely monochrome black-and-white environment because, say, she has a congenital condition that prevents her perceiving colour. Her vision is monochromatic, so for her everything appears like a black-and-white film. So Mary knows everything that can be stated in physical terms about the physical processes that are in any way relevant to colour vision, but Mary has never experienced colours other than black, white and shades of grey. Mary knows all there is to know about the neural basis of seeing something red, for example, but cannot see red herself.

It seems, then, that Mary has complete physical knowledge, but she does not have complete knowledge, for we can ask: if Mary suddenly sees colours one day, does she have a *fundamentally new* experience? Does she *learn* something new? The intuitive answer is yes. When she sees red for the first time she learns a new fact: *what it is like* to see red or that *it is like this* to see red. So there are facts over and above the physical facts, and since Mary's knowledge of brain mechanisms – all the material (physical) facts – is complete, the material facts are not all there is to conscious experience. Since even a *complete* neuroscience leaves out the facts of conscious experience, there must be something non-physical about conscious experience.

We can run the same argument for all sorts of conscious experiences including bodily sensations and emotional feelings. For instance, one may know everything there is to know about the neurophysiology of pain but, owing to some neurological condition, one may have never experienced the feeling of pain. Some people for instance, suffer from a rare, genetic disorder of the nervous system – congenital insensitivity to pain with anhidrosis (CIPA) – which prevents the sensation of pain, heat, cold and so on. Hence we can imagine Eddie, for instance, a future super neuroscientist, who knows all there is to know about the neurophysiology of pain but suffers from CIPA, as a result of which he has never experienced the feeling of pain. In addition, consider *Star Trek*'s Mr Spock and his memorable dialogue with Captain Kirk:

> Kirk: Have I ever mentioned you play a very irritating game of chess, Mr Spock?
> Spock: Irritating? Ah yes – one of your Earth emotions!

So when our super scientist is cured and no longer suffers from CIPA, and *feels* pain for the first time, does he learn something new (i.e. *what it is like* to be in pain or that *it is like this* to feel pain)? And when Spock is in love or frustrated for the first time, does he learn something new (i.e. *what it is like* to be in love/frustrated)? If so, then Jackson's argument seems to generalize over all our conscious experiences: the facts of our conscious experiences are over and above the physical facts.

There are two main general lines of response. First, it might be argued that Mary does not really learn a new *fact*; she is simply acquiring a new *ability*. To explain this objection, we must distinguish between two kinds of knowledge: propositional knowledge or knowledge-*that*, and knowledge-*how*. Propositional knowledge is factual knowledge (*that* something is the case), for instance, I may know *that* Paris is the capital of France or *that* the cat is on the mat. Knowledge-*how* involves the acquiring of abilities, for instance, one may know *how* to ride a bike or learn *how* to play the guitar. Now, it is suggested that to say that "Mary knows what it is like to see red" does not mean that "Mary knows *that* it is like *this* to see red" or that "Mary knows *that* red looks like *this*" (where "this" names the way that red appears to Mary). What Mary acquires are *new abilities*, not *new information*: she learns no information or facts that she did not previously know, but only abilities such as the ability *to identify* red objects as red, that is, to recognize them, and *to imagine* or *remember* having a red experience. This is no threat to a physicalist worldview. Physicists, for instance, may know all the relevant facts about how to shoot the ball in basketball but basketball teams are not desperately looking for physicists to staff their teams.[28]

However, it is not clear that *knowing what it is like* can be identified with having these abilities. Think, for instance, of the *moment* Mary sees the redness of red for the first time (fresh instance). That very moment, knowing what it is like to see red, cannot be identified with learning the ability to remember or imagine what it is like to see it, in that she is not *yet* able to remember it or imagine it. This further suggests that *knowing what it is like* is not to be equated with acquiring a recognitional capacity either, in that, plausibly enough, the latter seems to presuppose the former and therefore the former cannot be reduced to or be explained in terms of the latter. Consider, how is Mary able to recognize red objects, that is, what explains her capacity to identify red objects throughout different contexts after seeing the red patch? Plausibly, it is her knowledge of what red looks like. But if knowledge of what it is like is used to explain the recognitional capacity, then it cannot be identified or reduced to this capacity.

Second, it might be objected that the argument begs the question. Dennett (1991a), for instance, argues that Mary would not, in fact, learn something new because the premise that Mary knows all there is to know about the human brain and colour vision – even those theories that have not yet been discovered and formulated – includes, necessarily, a deep understanding of why and how the human brain is related to the experience of the redness of red. She would therefore *already know* exactly what to expect of seeing red, before leaving the room. Dennett's point is that the argument simply assumes what it is arguing for, that is, that no matter how much Mary knows in neuroscientific terms about colour vision, she will not be in a position to know what it is like to see the redness of red. But how do we know this? Although we may not currently have any conception of such a deep knowledge, it does not mean that such knowledge does not exist.[29]

What this thought experiment seems to establish, then, is that the proposition *that physical facts do not exhaust all the facts* cannot be known *a priori*, that is, without observation and scientific investigation. And the physicalist might respond that scientific investigation proceeds precisely by going out into the world; truths about the world are empirical truths, not *a priori*. Identities such as "matter is energy" and "water is H_2O" are *a posteriori* or empirical truths, established by experiment and observation; we did not come to know them *a priori*. Similarly, the identity "pain is C-fibre firing" is an *a posteriori* truth like the aforementioned ones.

However, Kripke (1980) disagrees. Although, according to him, some identities *are a posteriori*, psycho-neural identities such as "pain is C-fibre firing" are not. Kripke's *modal argument* against physicalism can be summarized as follows. Kripke starts with the notion of the identity relation: if *A is identical* to *B*, then *A is necessarily identical* to *B*. In other words, if *A* is identical to *B*, *A* is identical to *B* in every possible world: there is no possible situation in which *A* is not *B*. Consider again the case of water. Scientists discovered that the liquid we call "water" has a *particular* chemical make-up: it is made up of molecules that are themselves made up of atoms of hydrogen and oxygen. There is nothing more to being water other than being made of H_2O. The chemical structure H_2O *defines* water. So something is water *if and only if* it is H_2O. In other words, there is no possible world or situation in which one can exist without the other. Or consider the statement "The Evening Star is the Morning Star". This statement is necessarily true in that, as in the case of water, how can the Evening Star not be the Morning Star? There is no possible world in which the Morning Star exists, and not the Evening Star; since they are the same thing, the same heavenly body, the Evening Star will be there if the Morning Star is. So, then, if two things are identical, they must be necessarily identical.

Kripke suggests that the identity pain = C-fibre firing is not *necessarily* true and, hence, it is not true. For if this identity was necessarily true, it would be impossible for there to be pain without C-fibre firing. But it is possible for there to be pain without C-fibre firing. Therefore pain and C-fibre firing — as opposed to water and H_2O — cannot be one and the same thing. But how do we know that it is possible for there to be pain without C-fibre firing? Well, it is conceivable that there can be pain without C-fibre firing and vice versa: Descartes for instance, can imagine his mind existing without his body existing and Chalmers imagines the philosophical zombie, that is, a creature that is physically, functionally and behaviourally like us, but there is nothing it is like to be it: it cannot have any conscious experiences, so, for example, it cannot feel pain.

However, as we saw previously, the fact that a situation is conceivable does not mean that it is a genuine possibility. For instance, according to everything known in the fifth century BCE, there was no contradiction in thinking "matter ≠ energy" and "water ≠ H$_2$O". But as it turns out, these are not real possibilities. Similarly, a long time ago it would be conceivable to have heat (not the feeling of heat) without molecular kinetic energy. But now we know that there is nothing more to being heat other than being molecular kinetic energy, that is, the identity "heat = molecular kinetic energy" is a necessary identity. And a long time ago, one could easily imagine that the Morning Star could exist even if the Evening Star did not. But that is impossible. So although it is true that conceivability is our best guide to possibility, we should listen to Jackson's advice and be suspicious of giving intuitions about possibilities too big a place in determining what the world is like. All in all, we have not been provided with *a criterion* that would allow us to distinguish between our epistemic situation a few hundred years ago regarding such identity statements as "water = H$_2$O" and "heat = molecular kinetic energy", and our current situation regarding psycho-neural identity statements.

However, the *multiple realizability argument* casts some serious doubt on the idea that psycho-neural identities might be necessary empirical truths. According to this objection, there are indefinitely many physical structures that can *realize* or *instantiate* mental states. Since there are several pain-capable organisms (other than human beings), for example cats, birds and octopuses, and the physiological basis of a pain differs widely between species, then mental states, such as being in pain, for instance, cannot be identical to *any particular* brain state. If that is right, then one cannot identify a mental state type such as being in pain with a physical state type, such as a specific sort of brain state.[30]

To counter this objection, we might say in response that it is simply untrue that non-human animals have conscious experiences similar to our own. We might, for instance, complain that the objection is question-begging since it simply *presumes* that non-human animals have such experiences. Or we might wish to give an argument to the effect that they do not have similar experiences. Indeed, human conscious experience is a continuous procedure, a continuous going-on, which involves a world order conceptually organized by a self-conscious subject and a spatiotemporal form of awareness. As John McDowell points out:

> The objective world is present only to a self-conscious subject, a subject who can ascribe experiences to herself; it is only in the context of a subject's ability to ascribe experiences to herself that experiences can constitute awareness of the world … It is the spontaneity of the understanding, the power of conceptual thinking, that brings both the world and the self into view. Creatures without conceptual capacities lack self-consciousness and – this is part of the same package – experience of objective reality.   (1994: 114)

McDowell here seems to suggest that *what it is like* to undergo an experiential content cannot be the same for a non-self-conscious animal and for the self-conscious subject.[31] Now if you couple this with the idea that what it is like to undergo an experiential content is *essential* to it, then it follows that no content can be experienced both by self-conscious subjects and non-self-conscious beings. Let me explain, after some preliminary remarks. I take it that a "phenomenological state" is the *total way* that experience is for the subject at a time, the total way that an interval of experience is for a subject during that interval; a state in that sense would have *duration*. Constituents of a phenomenological state can be a patch of red, a trumpet-blast, an itch and so on. Now, the relation between the subject and his or her phenomenological state (or its constituents) is indicated by saying that the subject *undergoes* the state or its constituent. Further, phenomenological constituents may recur in different phenomenological states in the sense that different phenomenological states may contain tokens of the same constituent-type. Here, then, is what we might call the *phenomenological argument*:

> P1. What it is like to undergo a constituent of a phenomenological state is essential to it.
>
> P2. There is no phenomenological constituent C such that what it is like for a human to undergo C is what it is like for an animal to undergo C.
>
> Conclusion: No phenomenological constituent is undergone by both an animal and a human being.

In other words, no phenomenological constituent retains its identity across both animal and human experience, since what it is like for an animal to *undergo* it is not what it is like for a human to *undergo* it, and what it is like to undergo it is *essential* to it.[32]

As we shall see in the coming chapters, P1 is constitutive of the idea of phenomenology. Regarding P2, we can say this. In the case where say, a human being sees a green leaf he or she *instantaneously interprets it conceptually* (conceptualization or its mechanisms are always in use); a human being locates it spatially relative to other objects including himself or herself; a human being understands it as an object that persists through time, enters into causal relations; a human being sees the leaf through a penumbra of occurrent thoughts about other things – a human being may be reminded of the season, of the activities of squirrels, insects and birds, and so on. This suggests that what it is like to undergo an experiential content cannot be the same for a non-self-conscious animal and for the self-conscious subject.[33]

However, even if we can (tentatively) distinguish between "human pain" and "non-human pain", in such a way that each refers to a different *type* of a mental state, the type–type identity thesis must, at the very least, hold for "human pain", that is, there must be one-to-one correlations between human mental state types and human brain state/physical state types. Unfortunately, such type identifications have proved most difficult to establish empirically. L. F. Barrett (2006), for instance, observes that meta-analyses (Phan *et al.* 2002; Murphy *et al.* 2003) have failed to reveal reliable one-to-one correspondences or correlations between individual emotions and brain systems: different brain areas are implicated in the same emotion across studies and conditions (showing a lack of consistency), and different emotions often overlap, that is, have some brain areas in common (showing lack of uniqueness or specificity). Further, there is no agreement on the localization of emotions, such as, for example, anger and sadness.

In addition, switching to visual experience, the brain-identity theorist holds that a red patch in one's visual field, for instance, just is a physical property of a particular neurophysiological state in one's brain. But as V. G. Hardcastle (1995) correctly points out, it appears that there is nothing intrinsic in the brain that constitutes the difference between say, seeing red and seeing green. It appears, so to speak, that there is no neurophysiological difference between these two states; to the best of our neurophysiological knowledge, that is, there are no anatomical differences in cells in the visual cortices that correlate with colour differences. This seriously undermines the brain-identity theorist claim that each type of mental item is identical with some type of physical item in the brain.

1.4 FUNCTIONALISM

Functionalism descends from both behaviourism and brain-identity theory. Broadly speaking, functionalism comes in two varieties: *machine* functionalism and *causal-theoretical* functionalism. According to the first, we can think of the mind as a computational machine and mental states as functional states of the machine, whereas according to the latter, mental states are defined in terms of their causal role: the former identifies mental states with functional states, while the latter identifies mental states with the physical states that play the functional (causal) roles in question. Both allow for multiple realizability in that it is plain that the same functional state or the same causal role can be instantiated (realized) or played in different physical systems. For example, the primary function of the heart is to pump blood through the arteries and this can be done by a variety of diverse physical systems, that is, it is not necessary that whatever realizes or performs this function has to be a muscular organ about the size of a fist. The same function can be realized by a mechanical device implanted into the body. The functionalist then aims to abstract from neurophysiological details so that a wider variety of diverse systems can be said to instantiate similar mental properties.

Recall Armstrong's argument. According to Armstrong, pain, for instance, is an internal state of the organism that is normally caused by tissue damage and causes a certain pattern of behaviour such as wincing and groaning. Since neuroscience tells us that C-fibre firing is the internal state that is normally caused by tissue damage and that it causes a certain pattern of behaviour such as wincing and groaning, we should identify pain with C-fibre firing, that is, define pain as being the thing that plays a certain causal role. Armstrong saw his view as providing support for the brain-identity theory, not competing with it. In light of the multiple realizability objection, however, what is really important in Armstrong's argument is that the *internal state* in question is defined *functionally*, that is, as a *causal intermediary* between typical pain inputs (e.g. tissue damage) and typical pain outputs (e.g. wincing and groaning); it is that which is caused by certain sensory input and it causes certain behavioural output. This definition does not require that the causal intermediary be a *particular* neurophysiological state. The emphasis is given to the ability or capacity of the (internal) state to perform a certain function or fulfil a certain causal role, and, therefore, this state might be C-fibre firing in humans, a different physiological mechanism in a non-human animal, silicon painmakers and so on. What matters is that the state plays the causal role in question.

It should now be clear that there is a close affinity between behaviourism and brain-identity theory, on the one hand, and functionalism on the other in that sensory inputs, behavioural outputs as well as (internal) brain states are central to functionalism too. In this sense, functionalism is a more complete theory than its predecessors appealing to both observable patterns of behaviour and real-internal states/brain states of the organism to account for mentality. In contrast, behaviourism says nothing about internal states, and brain-identity theory identifies mental state types with particular physical state types of the brain. Furthermore, as opposed to both behaviourism and brain-identity theory, functionalism allows for multiple realizability: the machine functionalist for instance, defines a mental state as a particular functional state and it is plain that there are indefinitely many physical systems that can perform the same function, and the causal-theoretical functionalist takes a mental state to be *whatever* internal state performs the function in question.

In addition, according to the latter, for instance, what distinguishes say, a pain from a sensation of hot or cold is the distinctive input–output relation between these states. But the input–output relation includes not only the typical sensory inputs and behavioural outputs that are normally associated with each mental state, but also other mental states. This is a *holistic* approach to mentality. Pain, for instance, can cause not only, say, the emission of loud noises and escaping behaviour, but also distress, worry and so on. The latter are mental states that are on the output side of the pain input–output relation, and pain is on the input side of the input–output relation of distress and worry; the output of the last two might involve shallow breathing and brow-wrinkling, respectively.

So suppose you have a bad burn-pain as a result of touching a hot surface. The pain story in folk psychology or mental-state terms is this:

> your pain is caused by the hot surface, and pain causes distress and worry and the release of loud noises, and in turn, distress and worry cause shallow breathing and brow-wrinkling, respectively.

The pain story thus told contains a number of mental-state terms. These can be defined in various ways. One such way is to use the Ramsey–Lewis method (see e.g. Lewis 1972), that is, the idea that the claims of a scientific theory can be put in a sentence – the Ramsey sentence – and then be used to identify the entities that satisfy the theory. This method involves replacing all mental terms with *variables*, that is, x_1, x_2, x_3, …, meaning *there is something, there is something else, there is another thing not the same as any of the first two* and so on, respectively. We can then rephrase the pain story by replacing all mental terms in it with variables:

> There are an x_1, an x_2 and an x_3, and x_1 is caused by the hot surface, and x_1 causes x_2, x_3 and the release of loud noises, and in turn, x_2 and x_3 cause shallow breathing and brow-wrinkling, respectively.

This way we can keep the claims of the theory, withholding any ontological commitment: there is no specification as to what x_1 or x_2 or x_3 must be; anything can be x_1 or x_2 or x_3 as long as it can stand in the right sort of causal relation, that is, anything that can play the specified causal role. This way we can define "pain" by getting rid of all mental terms and without appealing to or specifying any *particular* (physical) states or processes (causal intermediaries) as follows:

> A person P is in pain when there are an x_1, an x_2 and an x_3, and x_1 is caused by a hot surface, and x_1 causes x_2 and x_3 and the release of loud noises, and in turn, x_2 and x_3 cause shallow breathing and brow-wrinkling, respectively, and P has (or is in) x_1.

Similarly, we can define "distress" and "worry". According to the functionalist, all our mental states can be defined this way and anything that finds itself in states that play those causal roles counts as having a mind.[34]

There are, in the main, two sources of trouble for functionalism. First, according to machine functionalism, a computer and I can both instantiate (realize) the same functional state in spite of being made of completely different material stuff. Indeed, functionalists strongly favour the possibility of artificial intelligence: the brain is analogous to computer hardware and mentality is analogous to a program (computer software) running on the computer. Mental processes are held to be algorithmic in nature, albeit very complex and sophisticated. On this view, the appropriately programmed computer *really is* a mind. As a result, mental content just is, or at least is determined by, the manipulation of purely formal symbols in accordance with syntactic rules.

However, it seems that there is more to mentality than pure syntactic manipulation of symbols. Here is Searle's Chinese room argument to the effect that programs that are defined purely formally or syntactically cannot constitute a mind:

> Suppose that I'm locked in a room and given a large batch of Chinese writing. Suppose furthermore (as is indeed the case) that I know no Chinese ... Now suppose further that after this first batch of Chinese writing I am given a second batch of Chinese script together with a set of rules for correlating the second batch with the first batch. The rules are in English, and I understand these rules ... They enable me to correlate one set of formal symbols with another set of formal symbols, and all that "formal" means here is that I can identify the symbols entirely by their shapes. Now suppose also that I am given a third batch of Chinese symbols together with some instructions, again in English, that enable me to correlate elements of this third batch with the first two batches, and these rules instruct me how to give back certain Chinese symbols with certain sorts of shapes in response to certain sorts of shapes given me in the third batch. (1980: 418)

From the perspective of someone outside the room, Searle's argument goes, once the person inside the room becomes familiar enough with the rules, the input–output relations are exactly the same as they would be if someone with a genuine understanding of Chinese were locked inside the room. According to Searle, this suggests that mentality is more than rule-governed syntactic manipulation of symbols "whatever purely formal principles you put into the computer, they will not be sufficient for understanding, since a human will be able to follow the formal principles without understanding anything" (*ibid.*: 419). So according to him, no amount of syntactic symbol-pushing or of syntactic processes (inputs and outputs, based on algorithms) can generate understanding or meaning and since mentality is not possible unless meanings are generated, no amount of syntactic processes can realize mentality. The mind cannot be a computer, no matter how complex.

Searle's argument raises important questions about the nature of meaning, especially about how meaning is generated from physical structures and processes in human brains. How do they do it? Searle thinks that brains, as opposed to computers, *do* generate meaning. But what we find in brains at a low level are just electrochemical processes, which in turn are just interactions between cells and molecules. So why is there such a difference *in kind* between biochemical processes in the brain and symbolic manipulation in computational processes? What more is to be found in the brain? What is so special about "the flux of ions in little bits of jelly": the neurons? In the same paper Searle considers the brain-simulator reply, which envisages a program implemented by the computer that simulates the actual sequence of neuron firings in the brain of a native Chinese speaker. Searle writes that "even getting close to the operation of the brain is still not sufficient to produce understanding" (*ibid.*: 421). But why not? Searle's less than fully satisfying general response is to insist that any artificial system capable of realizing minds would have to be able to duplicate the specific causal powers of brains, but it cannot do this *just* by running a formal program.[35]

Second, functionalism seems unable to account for the felt or sensed qualities of our experiences. It is generally held that some of our mental states are accompanied by felt qualities or *subjective feels*: there is something it is like *for us* to be in those states. Mental states with such qualities (or qualia) are, generally, our sensory and affective states. There is, for instance, something it is like for one to feel a sharp pain or an itch in one's finger as there is also something it is like for one to smell coffee brewing, or to see the vivid colours of a sunset. The worry here is that when we talk about our experiences, we focus on what it is like to have them, that is, on their distinctive qualitative character or subjective feel. When I have toothache, for instance, I focus on how it *feels* and it seems that a functional characterization of my toothache leaves out its qualitative aspect. In other words, it seems that a state can play its causal role even in the complete absence of its distinctive qualitative feel.

According to Nagel, "this inner aspect of pain [that it *feels* a certain way] and other conscious experiences cannot be adequately analysed in terms of any system of causal relations to physical stimuli and behaviour, however complicated" (1987: 36).

There are a number of thought experiments that are supposed to show that a state can play its causal role in the absence of its qualitative feel. I shall briefly look at the *inverted qualia* and the *absent qualia* hypotheses. The inverted qualia hypothesis runs as follows. Consider two people, Tom and John, who have inverted visual experiences (and notions) of the colours red and green. What is red to Tom is green to John and vice versa. When John looks at green objects, for instance, what it is like for him is the same as what it is like for Tom to look at red objects. Both have learned the meanings of colour words the usual way, and they apply the words correctly. Further, their non-linguistic behaviour is standard in every way. So, for instance, while Tom stops at a traffic light when it is red, John stops at a traffic light when it is green. Hence, the argument goes, Tom and John might be functionally equivalent, but subjectively different; in other words, two people who are functionally identical can undergo experiences that are qualitatively different.

According to the *absent qualia* hypothesis, it is conceivable that a system can be built, like an electromechanical robot, that is functionally (i.e. in terms of inputs and outputs) equivalent to humans and that completely lacks qualia (think of Searle's reply, for instance, to the brain-simulator objection above). So, for example, a robot can be programmed to *cry* and to *emit loud noises* whenever it is mechanically damaged, but we do not think that it *really feels* pain as we do. Thus, even if Searle's argument above does not succeed, *inverted qualia* and *absent qualia* thought experiments seem to show that functionalism does not account for *all possible* mental states, namely of the sort that possess qualia. And if a theory of mind must account for all possible mental states, and functionalism cannot, then functionalism is false.[36]

1.5 PROPERTY DUALISM OR NON-REDUCTIVE PHYSICALISM

I hope that our discussion so far has uncovered some of the most pertinent issues in contemporary philosophy of mind. Clearly, the problems of *mental causation* and *qualia* (or *subjective feels*) are among the most prominent. We have seen the serious difficulty for both the substance dualist in accounting for mental causation and the physicalist in explaining qualia in behavioural, neurophysiological or functional terms. Our discussion so far suggests that the following propositions have a strong intuitive appeal: mental properties are causally efficacious; mental properties cannot (currently) be explained in physical or functional terms; the physical domain is causally closed (principle of the causal closure of the physical). We saw that the views we have examined so far have considerable difficulty in accommodating all three and it seems that what is a serious problem for one view turns into another's advantage (e.g. mental causation is a problem for dualism but an advantage for the brain-identity theorist). Property dualism, however, claims that it can accommodate all three.

Recall that according to substance dualism, there are two kinds of substance in this world: mental and material (or physical). By "substance" we normally mean something that can exist independently, and have properties and enter into relations with other substances. (If something is a substance then it can exist in such a way as to stand in need of nothing beyond itself in order to exist.) Physicalists deny that there are two kinds of substance. According to them, there is only one kind of substance, namely physical substance, and all that exists in the world are bits of matter in space–time. There are, however, at least, two versions of physicalism: reductive and non-reductive (or property dualism). According to the former, there is one kind of substance, physical, and mental properties are *reductively identifiable* with physical properties, whereas according to the latter, there is one kind of substance, physical, but there are *two different kinds of properties*, mental and physical properties, and the former cannot be reduced, defined or explained in terms of the latter.

Non-reductive physicalism has gained popularity in recent years owing mainly to the idea that it can consistently hold all three claims stated above, that is, that the physical domain is causally closed, that the mental is irreducible to the physical and that the mental is causally efficacious. However, there are philosophers who deny this. Kim for instance, has provided a very influential argument against non-reductive physicalism on the grounds that the four claims below cannot be all true together:

(i)   A mind–body supervenience relation holds.
(ii) Mental properties are irreducible to physical properties.
(iii) Mental properties are causally efficacious.
(iv) The physical realm is causally closed.

Kim's argument is that assuming (i) is true, then one cannot consistently hold (ii), (iii) and (iv). The idea is that if mental properties are causally efficacious then either they must be identical to physical properties or there must be widespread overdetermination. The latter is not an option and hence the options for the non-reductive physicalist is either reject (ii) or reject (iii). In other words, the options are either *reduction*, that is, mental properties are identical to physical properties, or *causal inefficacy*, that is, mental properties are epiphenomenal. In the remainder of this section, I shall examine Kim's *causal exclusion* or *supervenience* argument in more detail.

According to the mind–body supervenience thesis (i), there is no mental difference without a physical difference. This implies that if two entities are physically indistinguishable then they are psychologically indistinguishable. So, for example, to say that pain *supervenes* on C-fibre firing is to say that C-fibre firing determines the *existence* and *character* of pain (you cannot stop being in pain *unless* you stop being in that brain state). A more precise formulation of (i) would read: whenever something instantiates mental property M (e.g. pain) there exists a physical property P (e.g. C-fibre firing) such that P determines the existence and the character of M; M cannot change unless P changes, and necessarily anything with P at a time has also M at that time.[37]

Supervenience is generally construed as an asymmetrical relation (as opposed to the identity relation): the mental is determined by or dependent on the physical, not the other way round. One of the advantages of this relation of dependency between the mental and the physical is its clear implication that the mental domain is anchored in the physical domain without at the same time implying physical reductionism: as we saw in §1.3, the supervenience relation states only a pattern of covariance between mental and physical properties and does not explain those correlations (why, for instance, C-fibre firing correlates with the sensation of pain). Thus supervenience is compatible with numerous doctrines in the philosophy of mind that are themselves incompatible, such as epiphenomenalism and brain-identity theory. However, although supervenience alone is not sufficient for physicalism, it is important in that it includes a claim of existential dependence of the mental on the physical. As Kim (2005) puts it, this does not mean that supervenience by itself brings the mental *close enough* to the physical. But it at least brings us somewhat closer.

Now, can we make the sense of the mental-to-physical causation given the supervenience assumption? Recall that the non-reductive physicalist holds that a mind–body supervenience relation exists (if it does not, then granting that (iii) is true would amount to rejecting (iv)), that the physical is irreducible to the mental and that the mental is causally efficacious. But, importantly, the physical domain is causally closed, so unless physical events are causally *overdetermined* the mental is causally inert. However, according to Kim, causal overdetermination (a case where a physical property P and a mental property M are *genuine* causes of P^*) is untenable. The physicalist, then, must choose between causal impotence and reduction (Figure 1.1). According to Kim, mind–body supervenience does hold, as does the *exclusion principle*,[38] and the physical domain is causally closed: "the conclusion is that causally efficacious mental phenomena must be reducible to physical ones" (*ibid.*: 153).

Thus, abandoning substance dualism in favour of property dualism and supervenience does not get us very far where mental causation is concerned.

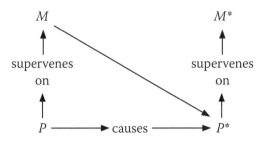

Figure 1.1 Although it seems to us that pain (M) causes the desire to get rid of pain (M^*), all causation takes place at the physical level where a certain brain state (P) is causally sufficient to give rise to another brain state (P^*). Since overdetermination is ruled out, M cannot cause P^* directly without violating the principle of causal closure of the physical. So M cannot cause P^*; P^* is only brought about because of P. Further, the M-to-M^* relation is ruled out: "in the case of supposed M–M^* causation, the situation is rather like a series of shadows cast by a moving car; there is no causal connection between the shadow of the car at one instant and its shadow an instant later" (Kim 1997: 286). Hence the most natural reading is that P causes P^*, and M supervenes on P and M^* supervenes on P^*. M only appears to cause M^* because both are instanced by the underlying physical events P and P^*. The M-to-M^* and M-to-P^* causal relations are only apparent, arising out of causal processes from P to P^*.

Arguments analogous to Kim's suggest that there really is no such thing as supervenient causation. In any situation in which the supervenience relation obtains, all the causal work is done by the physical or base properties alone. So this presents property dualism with a serious difficulty: if every physical event has a full explanation in terms of antecedent physical events, and if supervenient properties are not identical with physical properties, then it becomes impossible to see what causal work such supervenient properties can possibly do. Supervenient properties are thus merely epiphenomenal. The non-reductive physicalist, then, must choose between causal impotence and reduction.

Criticisms of Kim's argument generally revolve around the *drainage problem* (see e.g. Noordhof 1999). Critics object that Kim's claim that mental properties, as supervenient properties on physical properties, lose their causal efficacy to their subvenient-base properties is a general threat to all "higher-level" properties, that is, properties outside basic physics. This is why. Kim argues that all causal powers are contributed by physical properties. However, if one holds the exclusion principle and the principle of the causal closure of the physical, then arguments analogous to Kim's show that not only is there no mental causation, but there is no physiological causation, no molecular causation, only bottom-level physical causation (if there *is* a bottom level of physics, otherwise no causation at all). In other words, it appears that the supervenience argument *generalizes* beyond mind–body causation: since properties at the upper level are supervenient on lower-level properties, causation at any level gives way to causation at the next lower level. Causal powers seem to "drain away" all the way down to the fundamental level (downwards causal drainage). If that is right, then only microphysics could be the legitimate locus of causality, and all of the special sciences (e.g. chemistry, biology, neuroscience) refer to epiphenomenal properties.[39]

2. PHENOMENAL CONSCIOUSNESS

THE HARD PROBLEM

2.1 QUALIA

Imagine the best slice of pizza in the world: New York-style size, two thin and crispy crusts, with melted provolone and cheddar cheese, pizza sauce and toppings in between. Imagine you bite into the slice and taste its deliciousness. What is the underlying mechanism that enables you to taste the pizza? Contemporary neuroscience tells us that taste is a function of the central nervous system. It arises from the regions of the oral cavity and, in particular, from chemical changes in your taste buds, which are located on the upper surface of your tongue and the roof of your mouth. When these chemical changes occur, the taste receptor cells send information, that is electric signals, to the gustatory areas of the brain via a number of cranial nerves. This produces certain physical changes in that area of the brain and that enables you to taste the pizza.

Most people are not desperate to hear this story, although they might be desperate to taste the pizza. The taste of the pizza is one of the most familiar things in the world, but it is also one of the most mysterious. For *what* is *taste* and *where* is it? What magical thing happens when certain physical changes occur in the brain enabling you to taste the pizza? How can *taste* come as a result of nerve tissue excitation? It is incredibly hard to answer these questions. For as I argued in Chapter 1, it seems that even if a scientist scans your brain while eating the pizza, no matter how accurate the brain scanning is or whether he or she uses PET or fMRI scan, or even if the scientist uses a very advanced technique and painlessly cuts your brain open, he or she will not be able to spot the taste of pizza next to the grey mass of neurons. It seems that the taste is subjective, in the sense that it is not open to investigation from a third-person point of view. If so, then there is a real problem in accounting for the relation between the nerve tissue (objective property) and the taste (subjective property) that arises from its excitation.

The same considerations hold for all of our mental states that are accompanied by similar *subjective feels*: *felt* or *sensed* qualities. These qualities are typically called mental qualitative properties or *qualia* (singular quale) and are generally thought to be sensory or affective properties. Mental states that possess those properties are perceptual experiences such as those involved in *seeing* red or *tasting* liquor, bodily sensations such as *feeling* an itch and felt moods or emotions such as *feeling* elation, love or jealousy. In a preliminary way, we can define mental qualitative states by means of examples as follows: one is in a mental qualitative state if and only if one is in a sensory or perceptual state (including proprioception) that has such a qualitative property or one recalls or imagines such a property.[1]

As one might expect, there is currently a wide range of views as to the ontological status of qualia, extending from Chalmers's (1996) panprotopsychism (roughly the view that an experiential element is present in everything that exists) to Dennett's denial of the existence of qualia. Qualia have been paradigmatically seen as properties that are mental in the sense of being non-physical and non-physical in the sense of being essentially the objects of consciousness. In this sense, only non-physical properties can exemplify qualia. According to Chalmers (*ibid.*) for instance, a quale is an experiential or conscious item constituted out of the intrinsic natures of the fundamental physical entities. The intrinsic properties of the physical world include experiential or proto-experiential properties. Chalmers postulates experience as a fundamental property of physics alongside mass and charge and space–time. By contrast, according to Dennett, "despite what seems obvious at first blush, there simply are no qualia at all" (1991a: 520).[2]

There are also *relocationist* views. These are seen as middle-ground attempts to naturalize qualia or to oppose the long-standing traditional association of their qualitative and experiential character with the non-physical. With respect to qualia, relocationists attempt to move qualia out of the mind. According to one strain of this view, qualia are properties of external physical objects. Colour qualitative properties, for example, are moved all the way out on to the surface of the perceived physical objects (Dretske 1995; Tye 1995; Lycan 1996). So when one perceives a red rose, for instance, one is visually representing the actual redness of the rose. The represented redness of the rose is the actual redness of the rose itself. Thus redness is not a property of one's experience but an externally constituted property of the perceived physical object. Generally, on this view, qualia are not qualities of the experiences of, say, hearing, smelling and tasting, but rather qualities of public surfaces, sounds, odours and so on. In this sense, qualia are out there, in the external world.

The other strain moves qualia into the brain. This strain also has it that qualitative properties are not properties of the mind. A yellow or red patch in one's visual field, for instance, just is a physical property of a neurophysiological state in one's brain (Block & Stalnaker 1999). Both relocationist views are *reductivist* accounts of qualia: the former identifies qualia with externally constituted properties of the environment (representationalism), and the latter identifies qualia with physical goings on in one's brain (brain-identity theory). We have already seen some of the difficulties faced by the brain-identity theory. I shall have more to say about it in Chapter 5, where I shall also discuss Chalmers's panprotopsychism. I shall look at representationalism in Chapter 4. It is now time to move to the Nagelian notion of "what-it-is-likeness" and its relation with the notion of "qualia" and "phenomenal consciousness".

2.2 NAGELIAN WHAT-IT-IS-LIKENESS OR EXPERIENCE

Thomas Nagel (1974) famously provided the most influential characterization of the notion of "experience" or "consciousness". He wrote:

> The fact that an organism has conscious experience *at all* means, basically, that there is something it is like to be that organism … fundamentally an organism has conscious states if and only if there is something it is like to be that organism-something it is like for the organism. (1974: 435)

> [T]he facts of experience – [are] facts about what it is like *for* the experiencing organism. (*Ibid*.: 439)

This quote drives the point home. It points directly at "what-it-is-likeness", the salient but difficult to describe feature of a conscious state. I shall use the term "experience" to refer to the phenomenon of "what-it-is-likeness". If there is something it is like for one to be in a mental state then the state is experiential. If there is nothing it is like for one to be in that state it is not. Moreover, since "what-it-is-likeness" has been typically taken to be the hallmark of conscious state, experience is by definition conscious. In summary, then, I take there to be "something-it-is-like" for a subject if and only if the subject is having a (conscious) experiential state.

However, one needs to be careful here. To say that there is something it is like for one to be in an experiential state is not merely to mean that there is something that an experience is like. That there is something that an experience is like is a mere truism in that it is plain that there is nothing such that it is not like something. We can say, for instance, that there is something that a rock or a table is like. What-it-is-likeness in the Nagelian sense quoted above does not concern experiences or mental states as what-it-is-like concerns rocks or tables. Nagel says that "the fact that an organism has conscious experience at all means that *there is something it is like for the organism*". In other words, it means that there is something it is like to be us: the subject of a mental state. Hence "what-it-is-likeness" concerns the individual. If there is something it is like for the individual to be in a particular mental state then that state is experiential. What it is like to be in an experiential state is, in the relevant sense, what it is like *for one* to be in that state.

Sometimes the subject of the attribution of consciousness is the creature *per se*. We speak of a person or creature as being conscious or not. But as we have already seen, there are also cases in which the subject of the attribution is a particular mental state of the creature. David Rosenthal (1997) has suggested that "creature" consciousness is a characteristic that a creature has when it can sense its surroundings and is awake. (A creature lacks this kind of consciousness when it is in a dreamless sleep.) Whereas it is far from obvious whether the term "consciousness" is properly applied in this case, it is in "state" consciousness that the problem of experience lies.[3] State consciousness is ascribed to or withheld from particular mental states. We may say, then, following the current trend (after Nagel 1974) that one is in a conscious state of mind when there is something it is like for one to be in that state. Thus a conscious mental state is an experience; there is something it is like for one to be in that state. Of course, this does not explain what it takes for a mental state to be conscious. The most it provides us with is a distinguishing mark between conscious and unconscious states. Unconscious states are states such that there is nothing it is like for one to be in them. This distinction characterizes the phenomenon we wish to explain. We want to know what it takes for a mental state to be such that there is something it is like for one to be in it.

2.3 EXPERIENCE: THE HARD PROBLEM OF CONSCIOUSNESS

As we have seen, the problem of how physical processes give rise to experience is called the "hard problem" of consciousness (after Chalmers 1996). Why is it a *hard* problem? The major difficulty appears to be that the standard explanations in science are cast in objective terms (they are descriptive, given from a third-person perspective) but experience is subjective. So it appears that no description of one's conscious state in objective-scientific terms shows *why there is something it is like for one* to be in a mental state. Chalmers writes:

> *The really hard problem is the problem of experience* ... a subjective aspect ... It is undeniable that some organisms are subjects of experience. But the question of how it is that [organisms] are sub-

jects of experience is perplexing. Why is it that when our cognitive systems engage in visual and auditory information-processing, we have a visual or auditory experience? ... How can we explain why there is something it is like to entertain a mental image, or to experience an emotion? It is widely agreed that experience arises from a physical basis, but we have no good explanation of *why* and *how* it so arises. (1995: 201, emphasis added)

According to Chalmers (*ibid.*), there are easy problems of consciousness. These are problems that seem directly susceptible to the standard methods of cognitive science, whereby a phenomenon is explained in terms of computational or neural mechanisms. Thus the problem of the difference between wakefulness and sleep, the integration of information by a cognitive system and the ability to discriminate, categorize and react to environmental stimuli are such easy problems; there is no real issue as to whether these phenomena can be explained scientifically:

Why are the easy problems easy, and why is the hard problem hard? The easy problems are easy precisely because they concern the explanation of cognitive abilities and functions. To explain a cognitive function, we need only specify a mechanism that can perform the function. (*Ibid.*: 202)

On the other hand, there seems to be a real issue as to whether experience can be explained scientifically. A number of philosophers have recently proposed that the notion of "experience" does not map onto any of the current categories available in cognitive science and therefore it cannot be explained in cognitive terms (e.g. Levine 2001; McGinn 2004; Robinson 2004b). Nagel, for instance, writes:

[Experience] is not analyzable in terms of any explanatory system of functional states, or *intentional* states, since these could be ascribed to robots or automata that behaved like people though they experienced nothing. It is not analyzable in terms of the causal role of experiences in relation to typical human behaviour – for similar reasons. I do not deny that conscious mental states and events cause behavior, nor that they may be given functional characterizations. I deny only that *this kind of thing exhausts their analysis.* (1974: 435–6, emphasis added)

As it turns out, then, the main reason for claiming that experience cannot be explained scientifically is because explanation in this case needs to go beyond the explanation of cognitive abilities and functions.[4] The claim is that although such explanations can account for the easy problems of consciousness, they cannot fully account for the hard problem.

We saw previously that there is a real difficulty in defining experiential properties in physical and functional terms in that it seems, for instance, that a state can play its causal role even in the complete absence of experience, that is, there may nothing it is like for one to be in that state. There is a further claim here: we cannot exhaustively explain experience in terms of intentional or cognitive properties either. The alleged difference between the hard and the easy problems is precisely that the latter, but not the former, can be explained in terms of cognitive abilities and functions. By showing therefore that the hard problem can be fully accounted for in terms of cognitive abilities, we show in effect that both the easy problems and the hard problem have the same standing; if the easy problems can be explained scientifically then the hard problem can be explained scientifically too. And I think there is a way to soften the hard problem of consciousness. This is for later. Our immediate concern is to get a clearer grasp of the notion of "experience" and of the relation between the notions of "experience", "phenomenal consciousness" and "qualia" that have been the source of so much controversy in contemporary philosophy of mind.

2.4 PHENOMENAL CONSCIOUSNESS, EXPERIENCE AND QUALIA

To see more clearly why the phrase "there-is-something-it-is-like-for-one" or "what-it-is-likeness" has been the source of much controversy, we must appeal to Ned Block's (1995) much discussed attempt to clarify the concept of consciousness. Block has famously argued that the word "consciousness" connotes a number of different concepts and denotes a number of different phenomena. An important distinction he draws (and which many philosophers recognize) is between two different types of consciousness: *phenomenal* (P-consciousness) and *access* (A-consciousness). A-conscious states are conscious propositional attitudes, for example beliefs, judgements and desires. According to Block, although P-conscious states can be A-conscious too, they can occur independently of A-conscious states. Block suggests that both P-conscious and A-conscious states can occur independently of each other and they amount to different *kinds* of consciousness. The mark of A-conscious states is that they are available for use in reasoning and rationally guiding speech and action.

One needs to be careful here because the notion of A-consciousness is *dispositional*: not access but *accessibility* is required. The distinguishing mark of P-consciousness on the other hand, namely what makes a mental state phenomenally conscious, is that there is something it is like to be in that state. Block writes:

> P-consciousness is experience. P-conscious properties are experiential properties. P-conscious states are experiential states, that is, a state is P-conscious if it has experiential properties. The totality of the experiential properties of a state are "what it is like" to have it. Moving from synonyms to examples, we have P-conscious states when we see, hear, smell, taste and have pains. P-conscious properties include the experiential properties of sensations, feelings and perceptions, but I would also include thoughts, wants and emotions. But what is it about thoughts that makes them P-conscious? One possibility is that it is just a series of mental images or subvocalizations that make thoughts P-conscious. Another possibility is that the contents themselves have a P-conscious aspect independently of their vehicles. (1995: 230)[5]

Block is explicit in taking P-conscious properties to be distinct from any cognitive, intentional or functional properties. He explains that what he means by this is that P-conscious properties *do not essentially involve thought* or properties in virtue of which a representation or state is about something or properties definable in terms of a computer program.[6]

According to Block,

> There is such a thing as a P-conscious type or kind of state. For example the feel of pain is a P-conscious type − every pain must have that feel. But any particular token thought that is A-conscious at a given time could fail to be accessible at some other time, just as my car is accessible now, but will not be later when my wife has it ... The paradigm P-conscious states are sensations, whereas the paradigm A-conscious states are "propositional attitude" states like thoughts, beliefs and desires, states with representational content expressed by "that" clauses. (2002: 209)

Now, *prima facie*, there are some difficulties with Block's account. Block claims that the content of an A-conscious state is representational whereas the content of a P-conscious state is phenomenal (non-representational). But he emphasizes the fact that they interact. It is, however, hard to see how a P-conscious state can at the same time be a state with non-representational content, which can be used as a premise in reasoning.[7] Broadly, states with representational content are our beliefs and propositional attitudes. Roughly speaking, a certain content is representational if it has accuracy conditions, if it can, so to speak, be right or wrong, true or false. Representational content is the type of content that stands in logical relations. Block needs to explain how exactly the non-representational content of a P-conscious state can be used as a premise in reasoning, that is, he needs to provide an account of how exactly non-representational content can stand in logical relations. He says that the content of a P-conscious state may be *accessed in so far as* the content is *poised* for use as a premise in reasoning (representational). Thus P-conscious states *can* be A-conscious in so far as their content is poised for use as a premise in reasoning. But it is hard to see how this can be so since the content of a P-conscious state is non-representational. And, of course, it seems plain that the content of our experiences can be used as a premise in reasoning. At any rate, until such an account is given, there is a gap in Block's notion of P-consciousness.

Another difficulty for Block's account is his claim that P-consciousness can occur without A-consciousness and vice versa. One of the examples that Block (1995) employs in order to show that P-consciousness can occur without A-consciousness is George Sperling's (1960) well-known experiment. Sperling's classical experiment concerns what is called the determination of memory span. Memory span refers to the number of items (usually words or digits) that a person can hold in working memory. In the experiment, if a certain number of elements, nine letters in a square array for example, are briefly presented using a tachistoscope, it can be seen that the number of correct responses does not exceed four to five, regardless of the number of letters presented. There are cases where only three letters can be reported at a time. Now, according to Block, any three letters can be reported after the presentation of the array on command, but not all the letters, and therefore this is a case where all nine letters in a square array *are experienced*, but only three can be reported at a time. Block concludes that only three letter representations are *accessed*, and therefore P-consciousness of the nine letters occurs without A-consciousness of the nine letters. But recall that the notion of A-consciousness is dispositional. Not access, but accessibility is required. Therefore, it can be argued that all nine letter representations are A-conscious because each of the nine *was available for use* in reasoning and rationally guiding speech and action and therefore A-consciousness and P-consciousness (or experience in Block's terminology) occur together. Therefore, it is not at all clear that P-consciousness can occur without some kind of A-consciousness.[8]

Now, let us take a closer look at Block's notion of P-consciousness. Recall that Block says that a mental state is P-conscious only if it has experiential or phenomenal properties, the totality of which in turn are defined as what it is like to be in that state. So if a state is an experiential one, then there is something it is like to be in it and hence that state is P-conscious. But this characteristic falls short of providing the distinction between P-consciousness and other consciousnesses (e.g. a conscious propositional attitude – an A-conscious state in Block's terminology) that Block is hoping for. For one thing, *whenever* one is in a conscious state there must be something it is like for one to be in it. Imagine the case where someone discovers that his associate has lied about something or the case where someone suddenly realizes that she has lost her keys. In both cases the mental state he or she undergoes, in other words, the mental state he or she is in, is like something for him or her. There is something it is like for you to discover that your associate has lied to you and there is something it is like for you to realize that you have lost your keys. Are these P-conscious states? According to Block, they are. Why? Because there is something it is like to be in those states. These mental states, then, are experiences too. But then why should we maintain a distinction between P-conscious and A-conscious states such as conscious propositional attitudes in terms of what-it-is-likeness? Here is what Block says: "It is in virtue of its *phenomenal content* or the phenomenal aspect of its content that a state is P-conscious" (1995: 232, emphasis added). What Block says here is suggestive enough. A characterization of phenomenal content is a characterization of sensory appearances, namely how things look, feel, sound, taste and smell. The examples of P-conscious states that Block cites are perceptual or sensory states, such as when one "hears, smells and feels pain". So what is suggested by Block is that there is some kind of sensory quality somehow involved in the aforementioned mental states. And it is in virtue of the occurrence of such qualities that these mental states are experiences.

Although Block says that P-conscious properties include the experiential properties of emotions, beliefs and thoughts, we must notice that he clarifies what kind of experiential properties these are. He says that these can be "a series of mental images or sub vocalizations". Another possibility he says is that "the contents themselves have a P-conscious aspect" independently of their vehicles. As it turns out, then, there is a sensory quality or a *distinctive mental qualitative property* (a quale) somehow involved in all those states that count as P-conscious. The fact that there is something it is like for one to be in a mental state is cashed out in terms of the occurrence of some mental qualitative properties (or qualia) that are somehow involved in that state. According to Block, it is in virtue of the occurrence of such qualitative properties that we experience having a mental state. The qualitative mental state provides the what-it-is-like feature.

In this, Block is not alone. Chalmers has a similar conception of experience. He writes:

A mental state is conscious if it has a *qualitative feel* – an associated quality of experience. These *qualitative feels* are also known as phenomenal properties, or qualia for short. The problem of explaining these phenomenal properties is just the problem of explaining consciousness. This is the really hard part of the mind–body problem. (Chalmers 1996: 4, emphasis added)

[W]hat it *means* for a state to be phenomenal is for it to feel a certain way. (*Ibid.*: 12)

Hence, both Block and Chalmers identify experience with P-consciousness thereby claiming that the problem of experience is the problem of qualia. That is, what needs explaining is the problem of these qualitative feels, namely the properties involved in *tasting* some chocolate, *hearing* a sound, *seeing* a red patch, *feeling* an itch, *feeling* angry and so on.

Recall my two examples above: someone realizing that his associate has lied, and someone realizing that she has lost her keys. We said that in both cases there is something it is like for one to be in the corresponding mental states. According to both Block and Chalmers, whenever there is something it is like to be in a mental state, there is somehow some qualitative property involved. Would they, then, attempt to spell out the experiential aspect of these two cases in those terms? That is, would they argue that there are somehow some mental qualitative properties involved in those cases? I think they have to. The claim is that what it is like to be in a mental state is the totality of its experiential properties. According to Block and Chalmers, these in turn are qualitative feels, the associated qualities of the mental state. In their view, then, if a state has no qualitative feels or properties it does not have an experiential aspect; since the experiential aspect is missing there is nothing it is like for one to undergo that state. Thus if there is something it is like for someone to discover or realize that his associate has lied to him about something or someone to suddenly realize that she has lost her keys, then, somehow, some qualitative properties must be involved in those states.

This presents Block and Chalmers with some difficulty since they need to specify the qualitative properties that are involved in these cases, and the task of identifying those properties is, at the very least, a very difficult one. What is more, there is certainly circularity involved here since the what-it-is-like aspect of a P-conscious state is spelled out in terms of the qualitative or sensory properties involved and these, in turn, are spelled out in terms of what it is like to have them.[9] Block acknowledges this point when he writes:

Consciousness in the sense discussed is phenomenal consciousness. "What's that", you ask. There is no non circular definition to be offered; the best that can be done is the offering of synonyms, examples and one or another type of pointing to the phenomenon ... For example, I used as synonyms "subjective experience" and "what it is like to be us". In explaining phenomenal consciousness, one can also appeal to conscious properties or qualities, e.g. the ways things seem to us or immediate phenomenological qualities. Or one can appeal to examples: the ways things look or sound, the way pain feels and more generally the experiential properties of sensations, feelings and perceptual experiences [mental qualitative properties]. (1994: 210–11)

But whereas circular definitions are not as informative as we would wish, this is not the main problem with this account of experience. The claim that the problem of experience or what-it-is-likeness just is the problem of mental qualitative properties (phenomenal properties or qualia) is wrongheaded. The problem of experience or the so-called hard problem of consciousness concerns all phenomenally conscious and non-phenomenally conscious (non-P-conscious) states, that is, all mental states that are such that there is something it is like for one to be in them (independently of whether or not these states are qualitative). In a word, the problem of experience concerns *all conscious states*. Consider, for example, the case where someone realizes that the solution to a problem goes a certain way (Rosenthal 2006) or someone realizes that, say, the second premise of his recently published valid argument is in fact false. Plausibly enough, there will be something it is like for someone to have that realization. But no mental qualitative property need be involved in these cases. The fact that there is something it is like for one to be in such states shows that these states too are experienced. My past experience of cracking a mathematical proof can be different from my present experience. But *I am* experiencing these states all right, that is, there is something it is like for me to be in such states even if no qualitative property is involved. These states then, albeit not of the required (phenomenal) kind (since no qualia are involved), are experiences too, that is, there is something it is like for us to have them. Thus, it seems that non-P-conscious states, namely states in which no sensory or affective property (i.e. quale) is somehow involved are experiences too.

Yet it can be objected that a propositional attitude, for instance, is experienced because it is *accompanied* by mental images or sensory states. I might for example, suddenly realize the solution to a mathematical problem, and this might be accompanied by pain or elation.[10] Thus it might be argued that it is in virtue of the occurrence of such qualities that there is something it is like for me to be in those states. Peter Carruthers for instance, writes that "thoughts aren't phenomenally conscious *per se*. Our thoughts aren't *like* anything, in the relevant sense, except to the extent that they might be associated with visual or other images or emotional feelings, which will be phenomenally conscious by virtue of their quasi-sensory status" (2006: 306). So it may be urged that we have not yet shown that there really is no qualitative aspect somehow involved in those states.

There are two serious difficulties with this objection. First, as we shall see in the next section, there are other examples, which more strongly suggest that the occurrence of mental qualitative properties is *not necessary* for experience. Second, as we shall see in Chapter 3, there is good reason to think that mental qualitative properties are not invariably or essentially conscious. This means that the occurrence of mental qualitative properties is *not sufficient* for experience. Thus even if such states are accompanied by such qualities it does not follow that these states are experienced in virtue of the occurrence of these qualities. To this end, since mental qualitative properties are neither necessary nor sufficient for experience, we do not experience our mental states in virtue of the occurrence of these properties. And since the problem of experience involves identifying the properties in virtue of which there is something it is like for one to be in a mental state then the problem of experience is not the problem of mental qualitative properties (i.e. of sensory or affective properties that are typically called "phenomenal properties" or "qualia").

2.5 ARE THERE ANY PURE COGNITIVE EXPERIENCES?

Imagine two persons: a monoglot Frenchman, Jacques, and a monoglot Englishman, Jack, and then ask yourself whether the difference between them as they listen to the news in French really consists in the Frenchman's having a different experience. Galen Strawson (1994) correctly answers that Jacques's experience is utterly different from Jack's, even though there is a sense in which they both have the same aural experience as they are exposed to the same stream of sound. Strawson says that the difference between the two can be expressed by saying that Jacques, when exposed to the stream of sound, has an "experience (as) of understanding" or an "understanding-experience", while Jack does not. The point, as he puts it, is that "there is something it is like, experientially, to understand a sentence, spoken or read" (*ibid*.: 7). And this is distinct or additional to *hearing* or *seeing* the sentence.

Apart from cases such as reading and hearing others speak, understanding-experience occurs also when one thinks consciously. In this case, apprehension of conceptual content occurs, which has to be detailed in attempting to record one's experience as fully as possible. Understanding-experience is, then, an example of a pure cognitive experience (a conscious state devoid of mental qualitative properties) wherein:

the apprehension and understanding of cognitive content, considered just as such and independently of any accompaniments in any of the sensory-modality-based modes of imagination or mental representation, is part of experience, part of the flesh or content of experience … we need to allow that a particular case of understanding-experience can involve a specific cognitive experiential content while overcoming the tendency of the words "specific experiential content" to make us think only of distinctions like those found in sensory experience. (*Ibid.*: 12–13)

Notice that Strawson here argues explicitly for the possibility that experience and therefore the "what-it-is-like" aspect of some conscious states is independent of "any accompaniments in any of the sensory-modality-based modes of imagination or mental representation". Such modes of imagination would in some way or another imply the involvement of some qualitative property.[11]

Arthur Schopenhauer, in rejecting the picture theory of thinking, wrote in a similar fashion:

While another person is speaking, do we at once translate his speech into pictures of the imagination that spontaneously flash upon us and are arranged, linked, formed, and coloured according to the words that stream forth, and to their grammatical inflexions? What a tumult there would be in our heads while we listened to a speech or read a book! This is not what happens at all. The meaning of the speech is immediately grasped, accurately and clearly apprehended, without as a rule any conceptions of fancy being mixed up with it. ([1819] 1969: 39)

In addition, it is plain that there is an experiential difference between understanding what it is being said and hearing what is being said without being able to understand it (when one is exposed to the same stream of sound and there is no difference in the perception of phonemes). Thus, understanding-experience can be characterized independently of any qualitative character that a particular mental state may have. Mental qualitative properties, then, are not necessary for experience, that is, for a mental state to be such that there is something it is like for one to be in it.

It might still be objected that the what-it-is-like aspects of an experience of understanding derive largely from mental qualitative properties that accompany it. If that is right, then it is not clear whether or not mental qualitative properties are necessary for experience. Tye, for instance, writes that:

> We often "hear" an inner voice. Depending upon the content of the passage, we may also undergo a variety of emotions and feelings. We may feel tense, bored, excited, uneasy, angry. Once *all* these reactions are removed, together with the images of an inner voice and the visual sensations produced by reading, some would say (myself included) that no phenomenology [what-it-is-likeness] remains. (2007)

First, I must note that "understanding-experience" does not refer only to cases where one reads a certain passage or sentence. As Strawson puts it, it refers to there being "something it is like, experientially, to understand a sentence, spoken or read". And I am not sure just how Tye would account for the experiential difference between understanding what is being said and hearing what is being said without being able to understand it (when one is exposed to the same stream of sound). It certainly looks difficult to account for this difference in terms of being accompanied by a mental qualitative difference (or in terms of corresponding to any such difference for that matter). Second, as Tye himself notes, images and sensations are not always present in thought, nor are they essential to it. Take the case of *a priori* statements such as 5 + 7 = 12. What kind of mental qualitative property can account for the fact that there is something it is like for one to understand that statement?

Third, we could perhaps run a Chalmers-like conceivability argument. Let M be the proposition that there are mental qualitative properties and E the proposition that there are "understanding-experiences". It *is* conceivable that "M & $\neg E$". In other words, we cannot *deduce* that the subject has an understanding-experience by any number of mental qualitative properties. What it is like to understand is not reducible to any number of sensations, mental images and sub-vocalizations. It is perfectly conceivable that there is a planet full of creatures (the dim-zombies) that are able to have all sorts of mental qualitative states and yet they do not understand a thing. It is also perfectly conceivable that "E & $\neg M$". That is, it is conceivable that there are creatures (the straw-zombies) that are able to have understanding-experiences and yet they are not able to find themselves in any sort of a mental qualitative state. We might suggest then that "understanding-experience" stands over and above any number of mental qualitative properties and it is an experience in its own right.[12]

There are other examples of pure cognitive experiences. There is a general sense for instance, in which we experience our actions as *purposive. Agentive experiences* represent one's own behaviour as self-generated. Our sense (phenomenology) of self-agency typically includes the experience of authorship, the experience of mental causation, the experience of trying, the experience of decision-making and so on. As Daniel Wegner writes:

it seems to each of us that we have conscious will. It seems we have selves. It seems we have minds. It seems we are agents. It seems we cause what we do. Although it is sobering and ultimately accurate to call all this an illusion, it is a mistake to conclude that the illusion is trivial. On the contrary, the illusions piled atop mental causation are the building blocks of human psychology and social life.   (2002: 342)

It does seem that agentive experiences are pure cognitive experiences. And there do not seem to be any sort of mental qualitative properties that could account for the fact that there is something it is like for one to be in those states.

However, it is open to hold that whereas both P-conscious and non-P-conscious states are experiences (that there are qualitative non-cognitive experiences and non-qualitative cognitive experiences, respectively), P-conscious states are experiences of a different *kind*. There is a different kind of what-it-is-likeness involved in these kind of states and therefore experience is not amenable to the same explanatory account: the experiential aspect of a P-conscious state is different in *kind* from the experiential aspect of non-P-conscious state and therefore they are not subject to the same kind of explanatory account.

But why should we think that the experiential aspect of a P-conscious state is unlike the experiential aspect of a non-P-conscious state? What should be the motivation for distinguishing two modes of experience or consciousness, as distinct from different kinds of objects of consciousness? It is certainly true that what it is like for one to be in a visual conscious state is not the same as being in an auditory conscious state. This is because different modalities are involved and therefore different qualitative properties. But it appears that either there is something it is like for one to be in a particular mental state or there is not. In other words, either a mental state is experienced or it is not. After all, we do not distinguish a visual mode of consciousness from an auditory mode. We distinguish sights and sounds as objects of consciousness. One motivation would be that mental qualitative states are essentially conscious states, whereas beliefs for example, are not. That would be to think of the consciousness as intrinsic to its object, in contrast to the kind of consciousness involved in non-qualitative mental states, which is external to the mental state. So unless mental qualitative properties are themselves essentially conscious, we have no reason to believe that the experiential aspects of P-conscious and non-P-conscious states are not amenable to the same explanatory account.

Thus we should consider the possibility that the occurrence of mental qualitative properties is *sufficient* for consciousness. This is inextricably

63

related to the objection I raised earlier to the effect that a conscious propositional attitude, for instance, may be accompanied by mental images or sensory states, and this is why there is something it is like for one to be in it. This suggestion would have some force only if mental qualitative properties are sufficient for experience or only if they somehow carry consciousness within themselves. And this would, in turn, suggest that in fact we do experience our mental qualitative properties in virtue of their occurrence. This line of reasoning would eventually lead to the idea that whatever the story of the non-qualitative experiences may be, qualitative conscious states are a different story. For all we know, we might be dealing with two different kinds of experience.

However, as we shall shortly see (Chapters 3 and 4), mental qualitative properties are not invariably conscious; they may occur unconsciously and so are not essentially conscious. Thus even if such states are accompanied by qualitative properties, it does not follow that they are experienced in virtue of the occurrence of such qualities. This, in effect, removes the motivation for postulating different kinds of consciousness and leaves room for a unified account of consciousness: since mental qualitative properties are neither necessary nor sufficient for experience, and both P-conscious and non-P-conscious states are experiences, we can suggest that the same kind of experience is involved in both P-conscious and non-P-conscious states. Experience, then, must be specified independently of any qualitative properties and it is explanatorily irrelevant to such properties.

3. PHENOMENAL CONSCIOUSNESS AND THE "SUFFICIENCY" CLAIM

3.1 EXPERIENCE AND CONTEMPORARY NEUROSCIENCE

Once upon a time in philosophy, it was thought that one's knowledge of one's own current mental states is *infallible*. Thoughts, and mental states in general, were thought to be *transparent* to the thinker, that is, nothing can be in my mind without my knowing that it is there, whereas, say, my body is not transparent to me in the same sense. It was held that the mind is a totally transparent medium. If I believe that I am in pain, for example, then I am in pain, and if I believe that I am not in pain then I am not, and if a mental state occurs then I am aware that this mental state occurs.

However, Arthur Schopenhauer's and Sigmund Freud's work have revolutionized the way we think about the mind. "Mentality" is no longer synonymous with "consciousness". Freud, for instance, argued that people often experience thoughts and feelings that are so painful that they cannot bear them. According to him, these thoughts and feelings cannot be banished from the mind, but they can be banished from consciousness, hence constituting the unconscious. Independently of the degree of accuracy of Freud's theory of the unconscious, it is now commonplace that memories or repressed desires that are not subject to conscious control often affect conscious thoughts and behaviour. Propositional attitudes such as beliefs and desires need not be conscious. For instance, I have believed since childhood that 2 + 2 = 4, but only occasionally does it impinge on my conscious life.

More recently it has been recognized that perceptual states too need not be conscious. A competent motorist driving in undemanding conditions may ease her foot from the accelerator slightly as she sees the car ahead slow for the bend, but need not be conscious of seeing such, her attention being on the urgent conversation with her passenger on quite other matters. Or imagine, for instance, that you are driving too fast to identify some obstacle lying on your path, but you adeptly manage to avoid hitting it. Since you did not hit it you must have seen it (cases of peripheral vision provide similar examples). Therefore, mental states are not necessarily transparent to us.

Yet, according to most philosophers, although many types of mental states such as thoughts, desires and beliefs can occur unconsciously, our qualitative states or properties are *essentially* conscious. That is, if one is in a mental state with one of these properties then one is in a conscious state. Indeed, experience (or phenomenal consciousness) is generally construed as an intrinsic (in the sense of non-relational), atomic and unanalysable property. However, if you couple "atomic" or "simple" property with the claim that it is irreducibly *subjective* (as opposed to objective or to what is open to a third person – scientific explanation) then there is nothing to get hold of when trying to describe such a property. If "seeing something bluish" and "seeing something yellowish", for instance, are essentially conscious then experience is unanalysable and it is very unlikely that we could get any informative explanation of what their being conscious consists in. As Joseph Levine (2001) has put this point, experience construed thus cannot be explained since on this account the property of being conscious could not be given any articulated structure.

However, as we shall see in this chapter, we have little reason, if any, to hold on to this long-standing tradition. Recent empirical findings and philosophical thought experiments strongly suggest that mental qualitative properties are not essentially conscious and therefore their occurrence is not sufficient for experience. In other words, we do not experience our mental states in virtue of the occurrence of such qualities. If you couple this with the claim that they are not necessary for experience either, then experience must be specified independently of any qualitative properties and it is explanatorily irrelevant to any such properties. In other words, experience and qualitative properties are not amenable to the same explanatory account.

Let us take a closer look at our sensory states. Given that such states are paradigmatically qualitative, we can ask: can these states occur unconsciously? In other words, is there good empirical evidence for the distinction between conscious and unconscious perception? It appears that there is. Masked priming experiments, for instance, show that subjects see stimuli they are unaware of seeing. Although the subjects deny seeing the masked prime, it affects their subsequent behaviour and reasoning (Marcel 1983; Klinger & Greenwald 1995). Studies on blindsight (Weiskrantz 1986), visual-form agnosia and optic ataxia (Milner & Goodale 1995), change detection (Fernandez-Duque & Thornton 2000; Simons *et al.* 2002) and others provide similar examples. It is certainly true that arriving at the correct interpretation of such phenomena is far from easy, not least because of the terminological chaos in this area. "Awareness", for instance, a key term in those cases, is used in different contexts to mean different things. For a start, since to be aware or conscious of being in a particular state is defined in terms of there being something it is like *for one* to be in that state, in what follows I shall take lack of awareness to mean that there is nothing it is like *for one* to be in particular state with such and such features.[1]

Let us take each case in turn. Blindsight is referred to as an ability to respond appropriately to visual inputs while *lacking the feeling* of having seen them (while believing oneself not to be seeing them); in other words, when there is nothing it is like *for one* to undergo these states. The work of one of the pioneer investigators of the phenomenon (Weiskrantz 1986) and others (e.g. Stoerig 1996) suggests that the controversial and bizarre phenomenon of blindsight shows that one can perceive things visually even in the complete absence of visual awareness. Bindsight patients, in spite of being effectively blind because of brain damage, can generally carry out tasks that would appear to be impossible unless they could see the objects. For instance, they can reach out and grasp an object and they can accurately describe whether a stick is vertical or horizontal. More recently, it has been shown that blindsight patients are capable of some degree of colour discrimination and although they cannot recognize faces, they can correctly "guess" someone's expression (Stoerig & Cowey 1989). Blindsight patients, then, may lack visual consciousness or awareness yet they answer accurately questions about the shape, position and even colour of surrounding objects (despite being unaware of the visual information they possess, even when they use it).

It is most natural to think that this dissociation between unconscious and conscious processing in blindsight cases suggests that there are perceptual states that are not available to consciousness. It appears that blindsight patients lack a certain kind of access to the content of those states: even though, as it is believed, they process visual information, they seem to lack a certain kind of direct access to the visual modality or to the corresponding perceptual content. There are other similar cases. For example, patients who do not see anything on their right side, if asked to guess what is there, guess with considerable accuracy. These patients have some sort of lesion in area V1 of the visual cortex but possess unimpaired function in the other distinct areas that the retinal image projects to.[2]

Most recently, there has been reported a case of two patients who, although partially blind because of damage to one side of the brain, were able to sense and respond to emotions expressed by people in pictures presented to their blind sides (Abbott 2009). The patients, both from the United Kingdom, have the very rare condition known as partial cortical blindness. Their eyes are intact but they have damage to the visual cortex on one side of the brain. As a result, they cannot process information on the opposite side of their nose. Researchers found that the patients unconsciously twitched a facial muscle uniquely involved in smiling when a picture showed a happy person, and a muscle involved in frowning when the person depicted looked fearful (Tamietto *et al.* 2009). According to the scientists, the results show that our spontaneous tendency to synchronize our facial expressions with those of other people in face-to-face situations occurs even if we cannot *consciously* see them.[3]

Other researchers have also reported dissociations between aware and unaware performance. Diego Fernandez-Duque and Ian Thornton's (2000) work on change detection, for instance, has shown that changes in the environment can still affect performance even when they are not explicitly detected (see also Hollingworth & Henderson 2002; Hollingworth 2003). Another such case comes from Bruno Repp (2001). In his perceptual-motor synchronization task, participants tapped a key in synchrony with a sequence of auditory tones. In some trials, a change in tempo was introduced at a certain point of the sequence. Participants continued tapping until the end of the sequence, after which they reported whether they had noticed a change. For sequences in which participants reported being aware of the change, they made successful adjustments (phase corrections). But phase corrections occurred even in trials in which the participants failed to report the change. This is taken to suggest that awareness of change is not needed for such correction.[4]

David Milner and Melvyn Goodale's (1995) studies on visual-form agnosia and optic ataxia suggest that we have two complementary visual systems: vision for perception and vision for action. This proposal is based on a double dissociation between two kinds of disorder found in brain-lesioned human patients. Milner and Goodale's very influential theory of visual processing suggests that this functional distinction between our two complementary visual systems represents the anatomical distinction between the ventral and the dorsal stream in the visual system of primates. Only the ventral stream is directly associated with explicit conscious perception. Milner and Goodale (*ibid.*: 183) argue that only processing associated with the ventral stream results in perception associated with awareness, and that the dorsal stream normally operates in the absence of awareness. Consciousness thus appears to be a property of the ventral system and not of the dorsal system.

There are a number of findings that suggest this conclusion. Patients with visual-form agnosia have a lesion in the ventral stream and they cannot explicitly recognize objects or shapes and are capable of little (visually) conscious perception. They lose visual awareness of the shapes, sizes and orientations of objects. However, there is nothing wrong with their sensorimotor abilities. Despite their lack of awareness of the shape of objects, the patients had no apparent difficulty performing visually guided actions that require the processing of those very visual shapes. In other words, although they cannot explicitly recognize the shape of objects visually presented to them, they have no problem acting differentially with respect to those objects. The subjects can reach and grasp objects whose shapes, sizes and orientations they cannot visually recognize. While on the standard interpretation (Ungerleider & Mishkin 1982), the dorsal stream provides information about *where* the perceived object is, according to Milner and Goodale the dorsal stream does not just tell us where a perceived object is, but also tells us how to act bodily with respect to it. A natural way to explain these results is to say that the subjects lack awareness of their visual mental states.

On the other hand, patients with optic ataxia have a lesion in the dorsal stream and they cannot properly represent the size, shape and orientation of a target in a visuomotor transformation but can form appropriate visual percepts of objects by means of which they can explicitly recognize the shapes, sizes and orientations of objects.[5] The neurophysiological picture then suggests that there is a functional and even an anatomical difference between the sensorimotor perceptual system and the object recognition (conscious) system. Fang Fang and Sheng He (2005), in an attempt to provide a better understanding of how some patients can use object information without consciously perceiving the objects, have observed that in the visual system a ventral stream for conscious perception and a dorsal stream for unconscious perception are dissociable. In particular, both the ventral and the dorsal pathways contain object-sensitive areas. It was found that activation of the unconscious dorsal pathway is object specific in normal subjects, even when internocular suppression (binocular rivalry) had made them completely unaware of the objects being presented.

But there is more to it. While there is good evidence for the non-conscious nature of dorsal-stream processing, evidence suggests that substantial processing in the ventral stream also occurs in the absence of awareness, that is, unconsciously. On the standard interpretation (Ungerleider & Mishkin 1982), the ventral stream provides information about *what* the perceived object is. Although recent findings have shown that unless the relevant areas in the ventral pathway are active in visual agnostic patients, the processing of shape, size and orientation of an object will not yield visual awareness of those features, it appears that processing in the ventral stream is not sufficient for conscious perception (Kanwischer 2001). This suggests that one can not only unconsciously know *where* an object is and act accordingly, but also have all the information about *what* the perceived object is unconsciously.[6]

It appears, then, that perceptual states can occur unconsciously. Discrimination tests suggest that both unconscious and conscious perceptual states can represent sensible or perceptible features such as colour. It does seem that whatever distinguishes, say, red sensory states from blue sensory states is present even when the state is not conscious, that is, even if there is nothing it is like for one to be in that state. It seems, then, natural to describe these various subjects in mentalistic terms, as "seeing" the various properties of the objects, when explaining their accurate guessing or other discriminative behaviour, but without their being aware that they are so seeing. And the experimenters do so describe them, such descriptions feeding naturally into "psychological" explanations of the subjects' behaviour. Thus I do not see why we should not take such ascriptions of unconscious mental states as literally and realistically as we take ascriptions of conscious mental states in psychological explanations of ordinary behaviour.

However, some philosophers, following the Cartesian conception of mentality, have argued that one cannot separate being in a mental state from there being something it is like for one to be in that state. This view has it that all our mental states are necessarily conscious. Most recently, Galen Strawson (1994, 2005) has argued for this view. Strawson thinks that the entire range of our mental states, from pure cognitive to pure sensory, are conscious, with the proviso that "all experiential phenomena are occurent phenomena" (2005: 45). A mental episode, says Strawson, can occur only in a being that is capable of experience. However, he acknowledges that there are unconscious beliefs. But these are *contentless*. These are just belief dispositions and should not be properly counted as mental phenomena. Only *contentful* phenomena are experiential or conscious and therefore mental, according to him.

But it is not at all clear that our unconscious beliefs are just dispositions for beliefs to occur and are contentless. To say that mental states have content is to say, roughly, that we can describe them by specifying what they are *about*. Let us take, for instance, a paradigmatic mental state, an intentional state such as the propositional attitude "I believe that it is raining". The proposition itself – that "it is raining" – towards which one has an attitude is said to give the content to one's mental state. Now, are there any unconscious beliefs or desires that can be described in terms of specifying what they are about? Evidently there are. And evidently we can be wrong about the content of our beliefs and desires, and even the content of our perceptual experiences. There are cases where we act the way we do just because an unconscious desire has the content it has while we believe otherwise.[7] And since we *do* act in a certain way although unknowingly so, why still think that our desire to ϕ or *that p* is just a disposition and not a genuinely contentful (mental) state? Plausibly enough, my unconscious desire to ϕ or *that p* is (unknowingly to me) what caused me to do ϕ and it could not cause me to act thus if it were not an occurrent state.

There are many mental qualitative and non-qualitative occurrences that bear on the organism's moving about of which we are not conscious. In the cases discussed in this section, for instance, it does appear that our unconscious sensory states are indeed occurrent episodes and not simply dispositions for the occurrence of such episodes. As we have seen, there is a large amount of evidence that shows that our unconscious states have effects on behaviour and other mental states independently of whether the state is conscious or not. Of course, one way to account for these experiments is to say, for instance, that these subjects did not "see" the objects (in the sense that no sensory qualities [mental] have occurred) and therefore their actions are not amenable to a psychological explanation (folk psychological ascriptions). But this seems to be a rather counter-intuitive claim for both unconscious cognitive and sensory states. My unconscious desire to ϕ or *that p* can certainly be described by specifying what the desire is about. The proposition itself, namely, *that p*, towards which one has an attitude, gives the content to one's mental state. This means that my unconscious desire is a contentful (mental) state. And evidently it influences my behaviour and other mental states. Hence, it is an occurrent episode. Plausibly enough, the same considerations hold for our unconscious sensory states. It does seem counter-intuitive to say that in cases of peripheral vision, for instance, we can explain why the driver acts in a certain way (avoids the track) without appealing to the vocabulary of folk psychology. Indeed, how plausible is to say that the driver did not strictly speaking *see* the track? There does seem to be no sharp division between psychological and non-psychological explanation. Psychological explanation ends here.

3.2 BUILDING CONSCIOUSNESS INTO THE FIRST-ORDER VERBS OF PERCEPTION

I said above that one of the main reasons that experience appears unamenable to a scientific explanation is the mistaken assumption that the qualitative properties of our sensory experiences, such as a pain in one's finger, are *essentially* conscious, involving a different kind of consciousness: "phenomenal consciousness" (used interchangeably and uniquely identified with "experience"). In other words, some philosophers seem to think that mental qualitative properties somehow carry a unique kind of consciousness within themselves (i.e. Nagelian what-it-is-likeness). However, we saw in the previous chapter that there are non-qualitative conscious states that are such that there is something it is like for us to be in them, and in the previous section that there is overwhelming empirical evidence to the effect that sensory or affective properties are not essentially conscious, that is, there may be nothing it is like to have them. This suggests that the problem of experience is not the problem of mental qualitative properties (of the so-called "phenomenal" properties or "qualia") and that all the alleged distinction between phenomenal and non-phenomenal consciousness comes to is a distinction between the sorts of states that are conscious, not the kind of consciousness involved.

Here is a way to state these points more succinctly. (I shall use the following abbreviations: Q = mental qualitative; C = such that there is something it is like for one to be in a mental state, i.e. the state is an experience.)

1. Some Q states are C. [Terminological point: states that are Q and C are "*phenomenally* or *qualitatively* conscious" (PC)]
2. Not all Q states are C (e.g. blindsight etc.). [Hence: a state's being Q is not *sufficient* for it being C]
3. Some non-Q states are C (e.g. understanding, agentive experiences). [Hence: a state's being Q is not *necessary* for it being C] [Terminological point: states that are non-Q and C are "*non-phenomenally* or *non-qualitatively* conscious" (NPC)]
4. The difference between PC and NPC states is not a difference in the kind of consciousness they possess; it is a difference in the kind of states that possess a single kind of consciousness.

Since 2 is true and 3 is true, then 4 is true. The truth of 4 in effect removes the motivation for postulating different kinds of consciousness and leaves room for a unified account of consciousness. However, since the single kind of consciousness that is involved in both PC and NPC states has to do with what-it-is-like for a subject to be in the state in question, we might use "*experience*" to refer to this kind of consciousness. We can then be clear that the alleged distinction between "phenomenal" and "non-phenomenal" consciousness is *not* between *experience* and some other sort, even if there is some other sort. In other words, since both qualitative and non-qualitative conscious states are experiences in the sense that there is something it is like for one to be in them and the occurrence of mental qualitative properties is neither necessary nor sufficient for experience, we have good reason to believe that the same *fundamental kind* of experience is involved in both qualitative and non-qualitative conscious states.

Now, 4 being true makes the hard problem of consciousness easier, since it introduces the possibility that both PC and NPC are matters of cognitive abilities and functions: since both 2 and 3 are true, we do not experience our mental states in virtue of the occurrence of mental qualitative properties. What makes certain mental states such that there is something it is like for one to be in them has nothing to do with whether or not a certain mental state is qualitative. Following Rosenthal (1991, 2006), we can then suggest that to say that a mental state is an experience is to say that one is conscious *of* or aware *of* that state and to say that one is conscious of that state is to say that one has a distinct (higher-order) state, that is a higher-order thought (HOT), about this state. What it is like for one to be in a particular state is determined by the way that one's awareness or consciousness represents that

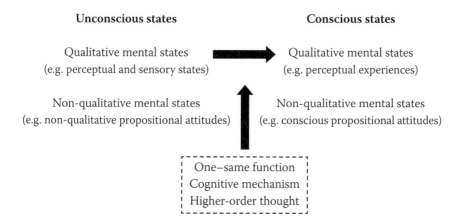

Unconscious states   **Conscious states**

Figure 3.1 All manner of (first-order) mental states can occur unconsciously, that is, can be such that there is nothing it is like to have them. It is in virtue of the same *cognitive ability* or function that there is something it is like for one to be in a mental state independently of whether or not that state is qualitative. This softens the hard problem of consciousness and puts it in the same category as the "easy" problems since, as Chalmers puts it, to explain a cognitive function we need only specify a mechanism that performs the function. Thus understood, experience is an aspect of cognition and of the brain processes active in cognition.

state. This awareness is explained in terms of one's having a suitable HOT about the (unconscious) first-order state. This way, a theory of *what it is to be conscious* is kept distinct from a theory of *what the objects of this consciousness* are. This leads us to divide philosophical labour and to characterize mental qualitative properties and experience independently of each other and employ different explanatory accounts for them (Figure 3.1).

More particularly, on this view, to say that a particular mental state is conscious is to say that I am *conscious* or *aware of* it, but my awareness of a mental state does not itself have to be something I am conscious of. The first-order state is experienced by virtue of my awareness of it, but this awareness need not be something I am aware of. But I can be aware of it (the second-order state) and that is roughly by virtue of a third-order state: further awareness to the effect that I am aware of being aware of a particular mental state. Hence, one can be in a conscious state (i.e. non-introspective) without being conscious of being in that state. To be conscious of being in that state would be to have introspective awareness of the consciousness of that state. For example, when one is in a conscious mental state – say one sees the cat on the mat – there is a higher-order mental state: one thinks oneself as seeing the cat on the mat. But only the first-order mental state need be a conscious state – there is something it is like to see the cat on the mat; the higher-order state need not be a conscious state – there need be nothing it is like to think oneself as seeing the cat on the mat.

It appears, then, that there is a distinction to be drawn between at least three kinds of states: unconscious states, non-introspectively conscious states (first-order experiences) and introspectively conscious states (higher-order experiences). We can use a small piece of notation here and say that if m is the first-order (unconscious) mental state then $A(m)$ is the non-introspectively conscious mental state, that is one is aware that one is in m, and $A(A(m))$ is the introspectively conscious state, that is one is aware that one is aware of being in m. Generally, it is a central commitment of HOT theories of consciousness that they provide a reductive account of consciousness. But how exactly such theories are reductive has not been explored in much detail. I shall formulate such an account in detail in Chapter 6, after I have more fully explained what the solution to the explanatory gap problem amounts to (Chapter 5) and examined a number of competing theories (Chapters 4, 5 & 6) thereby providing further motivation for this view.

Summing up our discussion in this chapter so far, there is good evidence that perceptual states can occur unconsciously. We saw that although blind-sight patients may see a cross on the paper, for instance, as evidenced by their regularly correct "guesses", there is nothing it is like for them to see it. The blindsight patient *sees* the cross on the paper, but not consciously. However, some may insist that the blindsighted patient only "sees" but does not see the cross, and that the driver "saw" the vehicle ahead slow, but did not see it, just because in each case the subject was not consciously seeing. This proposal seems to me to amount to an insistence that consciousness be built into the sense of "see", so that "consciously sees" is pleonastic. In itself this is just a matter of definition leading others to put quotes round my use of "see" where I do not. But if insisting on building consciousness into the first-order verbs of perception makes the problem of giving a naturalistic explanation of consciousness too hard, try the other way. Returning then to my sense of "seeing", whereby first-order perceptual and cognitive states do not imply consciousness, such states seem to me naturalistically explicable, at least in principle. Great strides have been made in devising first-order cognitive and perceptual architectures, and in identifying the cognitive and perceptual mechanisms of living things. Much remains to be done, of course, but there seems nothing here that defies naturalistic explanation so long as we do not suppose that first-order propositional attitudes and perceptual states themselves require consciousness, so long as we do not suppose that there is something it is like for that creature, in the proprietary – Nagelian – sense, to be that creature.

In the remaining sections of this chapter, I shall be looking at two versions of the "sufficiency" claim; namely, the idea that mental qualitative properties are *essentially* conscious (i.e. the rejection of premise 2 above). According to

Chalmers (1996), for instance, contrary to what the above findings suggest, mental qualitative properties cannot occur unconsciously, and according to Block (2001), they can, but nevertheless there is still something it is like to have them. In both cases, the idea is that the occurrence of such properties is sufficient for experience. However, this seems to fly in the face of the experimental evidence cited above. Blindsight patients, for instance, see the cross on the paper but there is nothing it is like for them to see it. And the driver saw the vehicle ahead slow but there was nothing it is like for him to see it. Why not? Why think otherwise? In what follows, I shall be arguing further for the following twofold claim: mental qualitative properties can occur unconsciously (*contra* Chalmers) but in the sense that there is nothing it is like for one to have them or, to put it differently, they are not experiences (*contra* Block).

3.3 EXPERIENCES *À LA* BLOCK

Block's account of experience is an exemplary case of the view that mental qualitative properties can occur unconsciously but that, nevertheless, there is something it is like to have them. Block allows that experiences can occur not only without one's knowing it, but even in cases in which one would firmly deny their occurrence. According to Block, in cases of visual extinction, for instance, where patients report that they do not see anything on one side of the visual field but if asked to guess what is there do so with considerable accuracy, subjects may be phenomenally conscious (i.e. in conscious qualitative states) but they do not know it or they are not aware that they are. Block argues that although subjects report having no (subjective) experience of certain visual stimuli on one side of the visual field, it is theoretically open to see these subjects as "really … hav[ing] phenomenal experience of those stimuli without knowing it" (2001: 203). He thinks that there is still something it is like to be in a particular mental state even if there is nothing it is like *for one* to be in that state. In other words, the state may still possess "what-it-is-likeness", even in the absence of subjectivity or even if one is not in any way aware of that state (without knowing it). According to Block, a mental qualitative state is *intrinsically* (non-relationally) and *essentially* conscious; the *seeing of a patch of red*, for instance, is an *experience*, awareness or "for oneness" is not required: there is something it is like to be in that particular state even if there is nothing it is like *for one* to be in that state.

In general, Block's idea is that experience can be attributed even to mental qualitative properties that cannot be reported; he thinks that states with such properties are conscious even if one is in no way conscious of them.[8] But let us have a closer look at some of these cases. In the case of visual extinction for instance, subjects presented with identical objects on both sides of their field of vision report seeing only one. Let us call the mental state that the subject is *aware of* and therefore able to report S. At the same time there is evidence that subjects are perceptually responsive to the stimulus they report not seeing. Let us call the mental state that subjects are *unaware of* undergoing S*.[9] Block (2001) takes this to be a case that shows that a state can be experiential even if we are not in any way aware of it. There is something it is like to be in S*, says Block, but there is nothing it is like *for the subject*. (Indeed, if one is not aware of what it is like, then there is nothing it is like for one.) He concludes that there can be experience (phenomenality or conscious qualitative properties) without awareness, that is, without one's being in any way aware of it.

But why should we agree with Block that a state can be experiential without thereby being anything it is like *for the subject* to be in it? Why should we take the extra step from "S* is qualitative" to "S* is conscious qualitative"? As I said at the beginning of Chapter 2, we should wish to distinguish between "there is something that X is like" from "there is something it is like for one to be in X". Recall that initially we said that the fact that we can experience things *at all* means that there is something it is like *for us* to be in the relevant mental states. Why should we then *assume* that although there is something it is like *for the subject* to be in S, there is also something it is like to be in S* but it is like nothing *for the subject*? And how could the latter have any contribution whatever to the *total experience* the subject undergoes at the time? It cannot, since S* can occur not only without one's knowing it, but even in cases in which one would firmly deny its occurrence (e.g. cases cited in §3.1). I fail to see how the phrase "what it is like to be in S*" can still have any theoretically interesting sense.[10]

In the case of visual extinction, the subjects may still be perceptually responsive to the stimulus they report not seeing but mere perceptual detection or discrimination is neither necessary nor sufficient for experience. Lack of responsiveness does not imply lack of experience and, conversely, lack of experience does not imply lack of responsiveness. It is a well-known fact that there are substances, such as curare (a muscle paralysant), that can produce imprisoned minds. In sufficient doses curare produces total paralysis. It is normally added to some anaesthetic mixes to keep surgery patients from moving. On regaining consciousness, the patients can feel pain but they may lose all capacity to express what they are feeling. On the other hand, perceptual responsiveness is not sufficient for experience. Imagine, for instance, that one is in a dreamless sleep and one moves in response to a muscle cramp. This is a clear case where sensory responsiveness is not sufficient for experience; there is nothing it is like for one to be in such a state. It appears, then, that we cannot appeal to any such perceptual responsiveness in order to account for experience since one can even imagine robots or plants being able to act accordingly. It does seem far more plausible to suggest that what cases such as visual extinction show is that even if there is nothing it is like for one to be in particular sensory states these must have occurred since one is responsive to stimuli one is completely unaware of seeing. Block gives no reason to suppose otherwise or that the states in question could be conscious in any other interesting sense of the term.

It is worth emphasizing that Block (1995) allows for the possibility that blindsight states be experiences or phenomenally conscious (P-conscious). He writes that the fallacy lies in "sliding from an obvious function of A-consciousness to a non-obvious function of P-consciousness" (*ibid.*: 232). Block claims that:

> it is a mistake to slide from a function of the machinery of A-consciousness to any function at all of P-consciousness ... the claim that P-consciousness is missing in blindsight is just an assumption. I decided to take the blindsight patient's word for his lack of P-consciousness of stimuli in the blind field. Maybe this assumption is mistaken ... if the assumption is wrong, if the blind-sight patient [does] have P-consciousness of stimuli in the blind field, then [only] A-consciousness of the stimuli in the blind field is missing, so [of course] we cannot draw the mentioned conclusion about the function of P-consciousness from blindsight.
>
> (*Ibid.*: 242)[11]

Block writes that "phenomenal consciousness is experience: what makes a state phenomenally conscious is that there is something it is like (Nagel 1974) to be in that state" (1995: 228). But Block's account of experience falls short of the full Nagelian formula in that "for oneness" is built into the full Nagelian formula, that is, the Nagelian what-it-is-likeness implies that there is something it is like *for one* to undergo the mental state: there is something it is like *for the subject*. So, following Block, we lose the element that makes this an intuitive characterization of consciousness. For any property *P*, mental or physical, there is something it is like to be *P*. There is, for instance, something it is like to be a tree, namely, to belong to a certain biological genus, there is something it is like to be a chair, and so on. But there is nothing it is like for the tree or chair to be a tree or a chair. Block is not taking a Nagelian characterization of consciousness *per se*.[12]

Summing up then, Block thinks that there is a sense of "what-it-is-like-ness" such that there is something it is like to be in an unconscious mental state. Undeniably, there is. But it is the sense in which there is something it is like to be a leaf on a tree; namely, being a leaf on a tree. This sense of "what-it-is-likeness" is not what Nagel was getting at, since it has nothing to do with the mind. This way we lose the element that makes this an intuitive characterization of consciousness. The notion of "what-it-is-likeness" as formulated by Nagel leaves no logical room for a sense of "what-it-is-likeness" that does have to do with the mind but leaves subjectivity out. That is, although we can form this concept of "what-it-is-likeness", it is a concept that has universal extension. An experience is a mental state such that there is something it is like *for one* to undergo it.[13] To conclude, it seems that are mental qualitative states of which we are not aware. If we are not aware of what it is like to be in those states, then there is nothing it is like for us to be in them. Consciousness is a matter of there being something it is like for the subject to be in the state in question. Therefore the mental qualitative states in question are not conscious.

3.4 EXPERIENCES *À LA* CHALMERS

As briefly noted, the other strand of the sufficiency claim holds that unconscious perceptual states, such as those described in §3.1, are devoid of qualitative properties. The claim seems to be that for such states to occur unconsciously is just for them to lack the qualitative property. On this view, "unconscious perception" means simply that "information" is available for use (to all or more usually part of the system), not that the same features that occur in conscious perception (*colour qualities* or *tastes* for instance) occur in unconscious perception. An exemplary case is Chalmers (1996).

In contrast with Block, Chalmers takes the Nagelian what-it-is-likeness to involve subjectivity or "for oneness". On his account, consciousness is always accompanied by subjectivity. In a more recent paper, Tim Bayne and Chalmers write:

> [W]hen a state is phenomenally conscious, being in that state involves some sort of subjective experience. *There is something it is like for me* to see the red book ... We can also say that *subjects* have phenomenal properties, characterising aspects of what it is like to be a subject at a given time. We can then say that a phenomenal state is an instantiation of such a property.
> (Bayne & Chalmers 2003: 29–30, emphasis added)

Elsewhere, he notes:

> [A] mental state is conscious if it has a qualitative feel – an associated quality of experience. These qualitative feels are also known as phenomenal properties, or qualia for short. The problem of

> explaining these phenomenal properties is just the problem of explaining consciousness. This is the really hard part of the mind–body problem. (1996: 4)

> [W]hat it means for a state to be phenomenal is for it to feel a certain way. ... in general, *a phenomenal feature of mind is characterized by what it is like for a subject to have that feature*.
> (*Ibid*.: 12, emphasis added)

Chalmers too takes "phenomenal" properties to be *non-relational* and *essential* properties of conscious states. These properties account for what it is like for a subject to be in those states. Phenomenal or mental qualitative properties (or qualia), then, are those properties in virtue of which there is something it is like for a subject to be in a mental state. Phenomenal properties, says Chalmers, deal with the first-person aspect of the mind.[14]

Chalmers's notion of "phenomenal properties" (another name for mental qualitative properties) is very close to the notion of the properties of Russellian sense data. The latter are mental as opposed to the physical (material) objects that cause them, and traditionally are taken to be the things that we directly perceive and sense, such as colours, sounds, hardness and so on. Mental qualitative properties would be the properties that perceptually appear to us, namely the qualities we seem to perceive things around us to have. These properties are possessed by mental objects – sense data – that cannot exist unperceived. On Chalmers's view, mental qualitative properties are directly and fully knowable by the subject.[15] It then becomes clear that such properties cannot occur unconsciously, that is, it cannot be the case that a subject finds himself or herself in mental qualitative states and there is nothing it is like for the subject to be in those states.[16] Since, according to Chalmers, mental qualitative properties somehow contain subjectivity or "for oneness", contrary to what has been suggested so far, unconscious perceptual states are not strictly speaking mental qualitative states. Mental qualitative properties do not really occur in states where there is nothing it is like for one to be in them.

Chalmers thinks that the qualitative properties of our mental states somehow carry subjectivity within them; a subjective *feel* accompanies their occurrence. As we saw, according to his characterization of phenomenally conscious states (conscious qualitative states), what it *means* for a state to be phenomenal is for it to *feel* a certain way. Blindsight patients, for instance, although having the ability to respond appropriately to visual inputs, are *lacking the feeling* of having seen them. These states, then, are characterized by the absence of any *qualitative feel*. These "qualitative feels", on Chalmers's account, appear to be another name for mental qualitative properties. The occurrence of a red qualitative property, for instance, has *ipso facto* a subjective feel. *Seeing red* is equated with (or defined as) there being something it is like for one to see it. Hence redness cannot occur or be registered unconsciously. Although I agree with Chalmers that there is nothing it is like to be in a blindsighted state, I find his view that qualitative properties cannot be registered unconsciously deeply counter-intuitive. Here is why.

Mental qualitative properties are the properties in virtue of which we distinguish among sensations. Each sensory modality corresponds to a distinctive set or family of mental qualitative properties. Discrimination tests suggest that the properties that correspond to each modality can occur unconsciously, since the occurrent properties (of the unconscious states) influence behaviour and other mental states. The fact that the subjects are *perceptually* responsive even though not aware of what they are seeing, as in blindsight, leaves, at the very least, logical room for postulating that a visual sensory quality that corresponds to that object *has* occurred. Dennett (1991b) offers an interesting case. Although he thinks that we cannot find a natural case of unconscious colour perception, he suggests an artificial one. A video game player, says Dennett, can learn to associate a certain flashing red spot with danger. We can imagine that the player's attention is distracted in such a way that if the red spot flashes the player is unable to report this fact. However, we may be able to gather evidence that "red spot" information has been acquired on the basis of a galvanic skin response (which provides a measure of anxiety).[17]

Another example comes from Rosenthal (1991). Rosenthal suggests that we normally speak of having the same headache all afternoon, even though the awareness of our pain is intermittent. Whereas the "headaching" quality endures all afternoon, says Rosenthal, sometimes we have a HOT towards it and sometimes not. Rosenthal concludes that during these intervals, that is, when we do not have a HOT towards the headache, there is nothing it is like to have it. And indeed, during these intervals we do not feel the hurtfulness of the pain. As Rosenthal puts the point:

> [W]hen one is intermittedly distracted from a headache or pain, it is natural to speak of having had a single, persistent pain or ache during the entire period. It would be odd to say that one had a sequence of brief, distinct, but qualitatively identical pains or aches. (*Ibid.*: 32)

It might be objected that the most that all these considerations can achieve is to leave logical room for the idea that mental qualitative properties can occur unconsciously. This might be less than entirely satisfactory in establishing the claim that unconscious qualitative properties are the same as our conscious qualitative properties except that there is something it is like for us having the latter. Why think that the same qualitative features that occur in conscious perception occur in unconscious perception? Because as opposed to claiming that those qualitative properties somehow, mysteriously, contain subjectivity within themselves, we can (intuitively) say that they can occur unconsciously – on a par with our other mental properties, such as beliefs and desires – thereby *explaining* those experimental findings cited earlier. We might argue as follows.

A good place to start is Chalmers's much debated zombie argument. Chalmers considers the possibility of a non-conscious creature, the philosophical zombie. The zombie is a non-conscious creature that is functionally and behaviourally indistinguishable from a conscious one. According to Chalmers, not only are such creatures conceivable but they are also (metaphysically) possible. Let P be the proposition that everything physical is as it actually is and Q the proposition that there are phenomenal properties (conscious qualitative properties). According to most philosophers, it is conceivable that $(P \& \neg Q)$. Since it is conceivable that $(P \& \neg Q)$, one can rightfully ask why, given that P is the case, is Q the case? Hence the explanatory gap; namely, there is no entailment from P to Q – one cannot *deduce* Q from P. But according to some philosophers (Chalmers 1996; Chalmers & Jackson 2001), from this *epistemic* gap one can infer an *ontological* gap: if we cannot deduce Q from P then we cannot explain phenomenal consciousness (used interchangeably with "experience" in their terminology) in terms of physical processes, and if we cannot explain it in terms of physical processes then phenomenal consciousness is not a physical process. Q is something over and above P. According to Chalmers, if $(P \& \neg Q)$ is conceivable it is (metaphysically) possible, and if it is metaphysically possible then consciousness does not supervene on physical facts. Since conceivability entails possibility, according to Chalmers, consciousness does not supervene on physical facts: two possible situations, for Chalmers, can be identical with respect to their physical properties while differing in their consciousness properties.[18]

Chalmers claims that zombies are possible and he agrees that what is conceivable is possible. Thus, Chalmers is committed to zombies being conceivable (we saw that Chalmers thinks that zombies *are* conceivable). What is conceivable in this sense, Chalmers claims, is what is consistent with natural laws. But what is consistent with natural laws is what is *explicable*. So zombies are conceivable only if their behaviour is, at least in outline, explicable. But the only explanation we can give of zombies' behaviour is in terms of sensory mental states (real qualitative states). Chalmers identifies sensory mental states with conscious states. Chalmers, therefore, can take this explanation *instrumentally*,[19] not *realistically*. But without a *realistic* explanation of the zombies' behaviour, at least in outline, we have not shown that zombies are conceivable and therefore not shown that zombies are possible. Alternatively, if we distinguish between sensory mental states and states of consciousness, we can allow that zombies *really* have sensory mental states. So *contra* Chalmers, our account can take explanations of zombie behaviour in terms of first-order sensory mental states *realistically*. So we can, at least in outline, explain zombie behaviour.[20]

Hence, since the zombie can detect perceptual differences and it can, so to speak, perceive the external world, it is indeed most natural to say that whatever distinguishes, say, red from green sensory states is present even when the state is not conscious. Therefore, although the zombie can see, hear and smell the world, there is nothing it is like for it to be in those perceptual states. The zombie, then, is a creature such that there is nothing it is like for it to undergo the detection of the real qualitative differences between the modalities and its reports. We saw that without a *realistic* explanation of the zombies' behaviour, at least in outline, one has not shown that zombies are conceivable (let alone possible). There is such an explanation. Plausibly, zombie-states are sensory states (i.e. unconscious qualitative states) and not sensory *experiences* (since the zombie is *ex hypothesi* unconscious). Therefore, it seems that there is something missing, something that would turn the qualitative *character* into a qualitative *feel*. Something needs to be added, then, in order to "light up" those states for there to be something it is like for one to be in them.

It is worth noting that we do not need to construct Cartesian thought experiments to discover zombie-like creatures or zombie-like behaviour. It appears that zombie-like behaviour is *physically* possible. An illustrative (although not uncontroversial) case is sleepwalking (somnambulism). Sleepwalking is a disorder characterized by walking or other activity while seemingly still asleep. While sleepwalking, some people may negotiate stairs, go outdoors or eat a snack. The subjects are performing actions without conscious control. It is striking that if the walker commits a criminal offence while asleep, the defence of automatism is available. There are cases where the criminal offender has not been found guilty because he was regarded as acting *automatically* – in absence of any conscious control.[21]

It is a common belief among neurologists that sleepwalking shows that that one can perform complex behaviour without conscious control. Now, what reason could we possibly have to deny that sleepwalkers find themselves in genuine qualitative states? Can we literally say that sleepwalkers do not really see, smell or hear anything? It does sound deeply counter-intuitive to say that they do not. One reason it is counter-intuitive is that, bereft of such ascriptions, we are without any explanation of their activities. At the same time, sleepwalking behaviour is a far cry from the sophisticated behaviour of the philosophical zombie. Sleepwalkers wake up enough to get the most primitive parts of the brain working: the emotional brain and the basic motor centres (without engaging the brain's more reflective and self-aware functions). According to William Dement, "in true sleepwalking, there will be some perception but not high-level cognition: Sleepwalkers are able to recognize a door but do not know how to get a door open" (1999: 211). It is natural, then, to suggest that sleepwalking is a case such that although sensory properties *are* registered – unconsciously – the fact that the subjects lack higher-level cognitive functions prevents them from *experiencing* those properties, that is, for there being something it is like for them to have those properties.

Moreover, considerations that show that sensory qualities are not invariably conscious can help us provide an informative account of how sensory qualities are to be distinguished from one another (since we cannot appeal to experience or what-it-is-likeness). Sensory qualities can be defined or individuated functionally, that is, in terms of their distinctive perceptual roles. In other words, since sensory qualities can play the same role independently of whether a creature is or is not conscious of them, then we can characterize them independently of experience. But if you identify sensory qualities with functional roles, then, bearing in mind that there is enough evidence that they can play the same role independently of whether or not the subject is conscious of them, it would be absurd to deny that they cannot occur unconsciously. This, in effect, seems to provide a good answer to spectrum inversion scenarios. Recall from Chapter 1 that the latter refer roughly to cases where functional duplicates might nonetheless have inverted colour-qualitative properties, thereby presenting one of the main objections to functionalism: the state might play its functional role in the absence of any sensory quality. On the inverted spectrum scenarios, what it is like for me to have sensations of red and green are inverted relative to what it is like for you. However, if sensory qualities can occur unconsciously then they can be defined in objective terms (by functional roles). And if sensory qualities are to be identified with functional roles, then spectrum inversion scenarios are not possible, since functional roles cannot be inverted. If that is right, there appears to be no intuitive reason to think that functionalism leaves open the possibility of spectrum inversion; cases where functional duplicates might nonetheless have inverted colour sensory qualities lose their intuitive force.

Sensory qualities and learning capacity

It is widely believed that acquiring new concepts generates new conscious sensory qualities. *Prima facie*, this seems right. For one thing, it appears that our perceptual experience becomes larger when we enlarge our conceptual capacities. Learning about music theory, for instance, enables us to hear chords differently and with more richness, and learning a bit more about gymnastics (or closer attention) enables us to see the gymnast's exercises differently and with more detail. Similar considerations hold with respect to wine tasting or to the appreciation of a work of art; the more rich our conceptual repertoire is, the more fine-grained are the differences among the qualities of our conscious sensory states.

As Rosenthal (2006) correctly notices, there are two ways to account for such a change in experiential content. It is either that "generates" means "creates" or "produces" in the sense that our learning of new concepts results in our perceptual or sensory states having qualitative properties they did not previously have, or that "generates" means that our new concepts result in new experiential properties by virtue of making us conscious of qualitative properties already inherent in our perceptual states. The latter means, of course, that the qualitative properties were present in those perceptual states before our concept learning and before our becoming conscious of those qualities.

Indeed, it is very hard to see how a concept can by itself give rise to a new sensory quality for instance. The cases of unconscious perception cited earlier seem to underline the intuitive idea that qualitative properties can be registered in unconscious perceptual states. It is most natural to suggest that the new concepts (or closer attention) can make us aware of sensory qualities already inherent in our mental states, rather than somehow create or produce these qualities by themselves. Chalmers's account, however, is committed to the view that the learning of new concepts can create new sensory qualities (since the latter cannot occur unconsciously) and therefore he ought to specify – at the very least – the mechanism by virtue of which our concepts can do this extraordinary task.

William Robinson (2004b) suggests the following mechanism. He urges that in order to acquire the fine-grained concepts for the qualities in our experience we undergo a period of training. In his view, changing one's concepts does not only change one's conceptual structure but also new neural connections are made in the course of the training process, which are not confined only to changing one's concepts. According to Robinson, this makes it perfectly possible that the connectivity of one's sensory apparatus changes. In this case, there would be "changes in the character of the sensory states themselves, and not merely in the conceptual apparatus by which one is able to connect one's sensory experience with classificatory and other behavioural activities" (*ibid*.: 104).

For one thing, however, this line of argument seems to over-exaggerate what the learning of a few concepts can do. It does not seem credible to suggest that, say, learning a bit about music theory can result in new neural connections, which, in turn, can "change the character of the sensory states themselves". For another, and pending experimental evidence, even if in some cases we require a certain amount of training in order to acquire the fine-grained concepts for the new qualities we experience, it seems far-fetched to straightforwardly deny that there are cases where this is far from being true. Sometimes in order to experience a new quality, it just takes one to try to listen more carefully or to just pay closer attention thereby simply applying the new concept to the (unaltered) content of her perceptual state. There are cases where the new quality is experienced immediately after learning the new word. This being so, we are left with the utterly unconvincing proposal, that concepts always mysteriously create new sensory qualities by themselves.

According to Robinson, however, there is another possibility for the way in which the training process may affect us. This is to give us the capabilities of attention that we did not previously have. He writes:

> If we have not learned to detect tannin reliably, putting the ques-tion to ourselves "How much tannin is in this wine?" may have very little effect upon us. After training, it may cause us to attend to tannin, and *that taste may then loom rather larger in our taste consciousness than before*. This change, however, is a change in the kind of experience we have. Allowing for it does not lead to the view that there are unconscious phenomenal qualities. Instead, it leads to the view that training can cause us to be capable of new kinds of experiences. (*Ibid.*: 105, emphasis added)

Robinson seems to suggest that allowing for the view that closer atten-tion enables us to experience new sensory qualities or the same sensory qualities differently, does not lead to the view that there are unconscious mental qualitative properties.[22] But this passage seems to give justice to the view that closer attention enables us to experience qualities *already inher-ent* in our sensory states: sometimes new qualities, sometimes the same qualities differently, maybe depending on our capabilities of attention. As Robinson himself notes, the taste of tannin may then "loom rather larger in our taste consciousness than before". There is nothing in what Robinson says here to suggest that a new concept always creates a new sensory quality by itself. Merely allowing for the possibility that closer attention can some-how produce new sensory states is not enough to reject the intuitive thesis that the learning of a new concept or closer attention may result in new experiential properties *by virtue* of making us conscious of qualitative prop-erties *already* inherent in our perceptual states. And since Chalmers has to deny this, there are further difficulties for his notion of mental qualitative properties.

The unity of consciousness

We saw in the previous sections that, according to Chalmers, mental qualitative properties are essentially conscious in the sense that there is something it is like *for one* to have them. On Chalmers's account, mental qualitative properties have subjectivity or *for oneness* built into them. Echoing Cartesian intuitions, Chalmers thinks that mental qualitative properties are themselves essentially conscious; they somehow carry subjectivity or *for oneness* within themselves. Thus they cannot occur unconsciously. However, this view is undermined by the zombie hypothesis, in that we saw that without a *realistic* explanation of the zombies' behaviour, one has not shown that zombies are conceivable (let alone possible). Further, appealing to cases of somnambulism, we saw that there is a need to appeal to the idea that mental qualitative properties can occur unconsciously in that for one thing, bereft of psychological ascriptions, we are without any explanation of the sleepwalkers' activities. Similarly with the empirical findings cited earlier. In addition, the idea that concepts always mysteriously create new sensory qualities by themselves sounds counter-intuitive. Hence, since explanatory power is a standard criterion by which (scientific) theories are evaluated we can conclude that our theory is better than Chalmers's in accounting for these phenomena.[23]

There are other difficulties for Chalmers's account. Our experiences are unified. They are underlined by what is commonly called a kind of "phenomenal unity". According to Bayne and Chalmers, two states are phenomenally unified when "they are jointly experienced: when there is something unified it is like to be in both states at once" (Bayne & Chalmers 2003: 29). The idea is that whenever a subject has at *t* multiple experiential states there is something it is like for the subject to be in all those states at once. Tye (2004) offers a good example. When a wine taster simultaneously tastes and visually perceives red wine, says Tye (we might perhaps add smells as well – admittedly tasting a glass of red wine when you have a cold is not the same as tasting it when you do not and it happens all the time and automatically), there are not two (or three for that matter) different or separate simultaneous experiences; they somehow combine to produce a new unified experience. There is something it is like for one to be in those three different qualitative states at once. There is something it is like for one to taste the wine or to experience all three states at once. As Tye points out, when at *t* one consciously tastes and sees (and plausibly smells) the red wine, one plausibly has one unified experience and not three single separated simultaneous experiences. There is something it is like for one to taste-see-smell the red wine.

Now, how plausible is to suggest that there are actually three experiences involved that combine into the total experience? How can we even separate the experience of smelling the wine from the experience of tasting it in terms of what it is like to have those experiences? Bayne and Chalmers write that "when A and B are phenomenally unified, there is not just something it is like to have each state individually: there is something it is like to have A and B together" (2003: 33). But it would certainly sound counter-intuitive to suggest that although all three different experiences are subsumed into one there can be still something it is like for one to experience them individually or that there is still something it is like for one to experience them individually in addition to there being something it is like for one to experience them together. What is it like to experience the taste of the morning coffee? Plausibly enough, one has a unified experience of tasting the coffee. One cannot still experience tasting the coffee independently of smelling it. And imagine that one tastes some red wine while walking barefooted along the beach kicking at the ocean waves listening to the sound they make and watching the gulls playing on the beach as the evening breeze blows warm and dry. How can we account for this unified experience? How many little experiences occur simultaneously (to combine the unified or total experience), and can be separated and accounted for in terms of what it is like to have them? In other words, what are the conjuncts of this conjunction? It is not clear how we can even begin to differentiate this unified experiential state into atomic experiences. The same considerations apply to one's concert experience. How are we to separate this experience into little experiences? How can there still be something to experience every mental qualitative property registered in our mental states? Does every little sound count? As Schopenhauer would put it: what a tumult there would be in our heads while we listened to a rock concert!

This is not what happens at all. What one has is, in Searle's phrase, "a single, unified conscious field containing visual, auditory and other aspects" (2002: 55). When one is at a concert one has a single, unified, structured experience. It is indeed most natural to suggest that having a higher-order state, that is, a thought about these qualitative states, "smoothes them out" (in Rosenthal's phrase) so that they are not experienced as particulate or discontinuous but rather as ultimately homogeneous and unified. One finds oneself in a single experiential state and what it is like for one to be in such a state is determined by one's awareness of it, namely by the way one's HOT represents oneself as having it, not by the mental qualitative properties themselves. In other words, the subject is aware of being in a sensory state with such and such mental qualitative properties and not with such and such experiences. The unified experience is not the totality of little experiences but a single experience that has such and such qualitative properties.

Immanuel Kant famously argued that prior to *synthesis*[24] and conceptual organization, a manifold of intuitions[25] would be an undifferentiated buzzing confusion. That is to say, the information received by the senses needs organizing. But how is it that our particular sensory qualities of our sensations result in the remarkable homogeneity of our experiences? Here is how Wilfrid Sellars illustrates the point:

> The manifest ice cube presents itself to us as something which is pink through and through, as a pink continuum, all the regions of which, however small, are pink. It presents itself to us as *ultimately homogeneous*; and an ice cube variegated in colour is, though not homogeneous in its specific colour, "ultimately homogeneous", in the sense to which I am calling attention, with respect to the generic trait of being coloured. (1963: 26)

Sellars's point may seem to raise a problem for an identity physicalist account, that is, the idea that experiences are identical with physical or neurophysiological states. The point is that it is difficult to see how the occurrence of a smooth continuous expanse of a certain colour of an object in our visual experience can be identical with a brain process that must involve particulate, discontinuous affairs such as transfers of or interactions among large numbers of electrons. Being smooth is a structural property, and being particulate or discontinuous is also a structural property. But this suggests that at least some mental events exemplify structural properties that are not exemplified by any brain event. Hence, it follows that the mental event and the brain event do not share all of their (structural) properties and therefore they cannot be identical. However, the point of interest here is this. Without getting into too much detail, following Kant, we can suggest that concepts must be applied to sensory states in order to organize sensory information into a coherent array of objects. So we experience this information as homogeneous in the way Sellars illustrated because that is the way that we are conscious of these states. Having a belief about these states smoothes them out so that they are not experienced as particulate or discontinuous but rather as ultimately homogeneous.

Now, recall the example where one tastes some wine on the beach. As is widely agreed, consciousness appears to be highly fragmented with manifold streams of perceptual content processed in parallel in different regions of the brain (Dennett 1991b). There is no stage at which all these contents are integrated into a conscious manifold (experiential state). Contents appear to become experienced on a piecemeal basis and not all at once. Immediately related is the phenomenon of shifts in attention. There are sensory states that are conscious only some of the time. Instead of thinking that sensory states are persistent and conscious all the time, it seems more likely that through shift in attention – the target of one's HOT is different – only some sensory states are conscious, and for only some of the time.[26] This fits well with the idea that what makes a mental state conscious is an *occurrent episode* and not merely a *dispositional thought*. Contents "light up" subjectively, as Rosenthal would put it, on a piecemeal basis by virtue of having a HOT to the effect that one is in the state with such and such qualitative content (of course, content need not necessarily be qualitative).[27]

Moreover, the phenomenon of "change blindness" seems to give justice to the idea that the qualitative aspect of the state that one is in diverges from the HOT account is true. Change blindness refers to the inability to detect what should be obvious changes in a (visual) scene. Very large changes may occur in full view in a visual scene (in visual perception) that are not noticed. A number of studies have shown that under certain circumstances very large changes can be made in a visual scene without observers noticing them. A change, which occupies in a very large portion of the visual field, may not be noticed if it is not part of what would be normally said about the picture: in other words, if it is classified as insignificant or of marginal interest. These findings appear to suggest that although observers have the impression that they experience every little detail they see in the picture they are presented with, in fact, they can notice or are able to report a limited range of information. It appears that there is a kind of attentional "bottleneck", which limits information transfer into memory, that is, only a fraction of the information available in a scene is transferred into visual storage for later report or comparison. An example is the case of inattentional blindness. Arien Mack and Irvin Rock (1998), for instance, used a task where observers performed an attention-demanding visual task. At a given moment, a large, unexpected visual event took place. Even though such an event would be totally obvious under normal circumstances, and even though the event takes place in full view, it was often not noticed.[28]

Finally, we can ask: what is the *unification principle*? In other words, what makes it the case that instead of (or in addition to?) tasting and seeing and smelling the red wine, one is having a *unified experience* of tasting-seeing-smelling it, thereby being something it is like for one to taste-see-smell the red wine? What *explains* why, instead of having an experiential tumult in our heads when we are at a concert, we have smooth unified experience? Is it another intrinsic property of the (allegedly) essentially conscious mental qualitative states? In Bayne and Chalmers's view, it seems that it just happens that one is having a unified experience: it is a happy coincidence. However, appealing to a HOT account of experience we can give an *explanation* of why it is that when one is at a concert, for instance, one has a unified and structured experience. It is indeed plausible to suggest that having a HOT about these qualitative states smoothes them out so that they are not experienced as particulate or sporadic but rather as ultimately homogeneous and unified. This is further supported by the idea that contents are experienced on a piecemeal basis (not all at once) and by the phenomenon of shifts in attention.

3.5 SUMMING UP

We saw in this chapter that not only is it open to hold that mental qualitative properties can be registered in unconscious states – without being experienced – but also that there is good reason for this. Although there are serious objections to Chalmers's notion of mental qualitative properties (or "phenomenal" properties or "qualia"), there are no such difficulties for an account that construes experience independently of any qualitative properties. We shall see in Chapter 5 that there are further problems with Chalmers's dualist account. Most importantly, Chalmers's account leaves a wide-open explanatory gap. And, arguably, ontological dualism is too high a price to pay for an account that lacks in explanatory force.

Now, allowing that mental qualitative properties can occur unconsciously and bearing in mind that there is nothing it is like for one to have these properties, we can conclude that mental qualitative properties are not *sufficient* for experience. And since mental qualitative properties are not *necessary* for experience either, we do not experience our mental states by virtue of the occurrence of such properties. Something needs to be added on.

It has been suggested that the additional element is a certain *dispositional role* played by the first-order mental state. Since the question we are dealing with is what distinguishes non-experiences from (first-order) experiences (or non-introspectively conscious states), it may be urged that first-order experiences are such that there is something it is like for one to be in them because they are disposed to bring about higher-order states such as conscious thoughts and beliefs. On this account, a non-introspectively conscious state is such that there is something it is like for one to be in it because it is somehow disposed to bring about introspectively conscious states. The idea is that no occurrent higher-order state is required for first-order experiences. According to the dispositionalist view, first-order experiences are first-order states that meet certain conditions; most importantly, they are *disposed* or *poised* to bring about introspectively conscious states, or, in other words, to have a direct impact on the subject's belief system.

In this view, then, there is an extra element (e.g. manner of representation or dispositional role) that makes our mental qualitative states conscious. On this account, all mental qualitative states that meet certain specifiable conditions are conscious; no further awareness or a distinct state about them need occur. But since those mental states that meet these conditions are invariably conscious, the occurrence of a *certain kind* of first-order mental qualitative state is *sufficient* for experience. Thus we have not yet shown that all manner of first-order mental states (qualitative or not) can occur unconsciously and that experience must be specified independently of any mental qualitative states or properties.

In the following chapter (Chapter 4), I shall argue that first-order states cannot be experienced without the *occurrence* of a distinct higher-order state. In other words, what makes a mental state conscious must be an occurrent thought, not merely a disposition for this thought to occur. More support for a cognitive theory of experience will come from Chapter 5, where I shall show the limitations of neuroscience. It will appear that we cannot explain experience in other than cognitive terms. In the last chapter, I shall show why a higher-order-thought view is preferable to a higher-order-perception view and I shall specify more exactly how it can help us solve the hard problem of consciousness or close the explanatory gap.

4. EXPERIENCE AND FIRST-ORDER REPRESENTATIONALISM

4.1 INTENTIONALITY, EXPERIENCE AND REPRESENTATIONALISM

According to dispositionalists, we experience our first-order states by virtue of a certain kind of *dispositional role* that these states have. Dispositionalists claim that no higher-order state is required for a first-order state to be *actually* conscious, but only the potential to generate a higher-order state. According to the dispositionalist view, first-order experiences are first-order states that meet certain conditions. On this account, there is still a necessary tie between mental qualitative properties and experience. But it appears that there is a difference between such accounts and accounts such as those of Block and Chalmers. With respect to our sensory states, for example, according to the dispositionalists there is an extra element (i.e. a dispositional role functionally defined) that makes our sensory states conscious. On this view, one can still maintain that whereas no distinct higher-order state is necessary for first-order experiences, there is still a distinction to be made between conscious and unconscious sensory qualities. In other words, not all qualitative states possess Nagelian "what-it-is-likeness": they must meet certain specifiable conditions.

In this chapter, I shall consider the dispositionalist approach to experience. Since these dispositionalist accounts are typically intentionalist or representationalist, I shall start my discussion by making a few remarks on the relation between the notion of intentionality and contemporary representationalism. Representationalism should not be confused with the traditional representational theory of perception, according to which we perceive physical objects and properties indirectly in virtue of being directly aware of some sensory or mental items that represent the physical objects and their properties. According to this traditional representational theory of perception, the world we see in perceptual experience is not the real external world itself, but merely a miniature virtual-reality replica of that world (an internal representation). The realist variant of this view is that we are directly aware of, or in direct contact with, intermediate mental objects that represent and are caused by physical objects. This view is called indirect realism. The main rival view is called direct or naive realism and maintains that we perceive the world directly and not in virtue of being aware of intermediaries, such as images, ideas, sense impressions, sensations and so forth.

Generally, according to modern representationalism, perceptual experiences are representational – they carry intentional content – but they do not involve indirect realism, that is, they do not encompass the main doctrine of the traditional representational theory of perception that we are not in direct or immediate contact with the external world. Representational states are involved in perception, but neither they nor any of their components involve objects, images or any sort of intermediaries that constitute a veil between the subject and the world. Hence representationalism in the contemporary philosophy of mind is a form of direct realism.

The idea of representation has been central in discussions of intentionality for many years and recently begun to play a wider role in the philosophy of mind, in particular, in theories of consciousness. Generally, problems of consciousness are generally thought to be less tractable than those of intentionality. The aim of representationalist theories of consciousness is to extend the treatment of intentionality to that of consciousness, thereby showing that if intentionality is well understood in representational terms, then so can be the phenomena of consciousness. Let us look more closely at the link between conscious mental states and intentionality.

Some 100 years ago, Franz Brentano claimed that intentionality is the "mark of the mental".[1] One way of explaining what is meant by intentionality in the philosophical sense is to say that it is the aspect of mental states that consists in their being of or about things. Intentionality is the directedness of the mind. Mental states have, or are directed towards, some object or other. Mental states have an *aboutness* in that they are about something or other. If you are thinking about Rome or about your meeting with the dentist tomorrow then your thinking is directed towards (or is about) Rome or your meeting with the dentist. Furthermore, we have the ability to believe in, think of and even worship nonexistent things (e.g. Superman or the Flying Spaghetti Monster). We cannot cut a nonexistent piece of paper or be to the left of a nonexistent chair. The idea, generally, is that thinking of some*thing* does not entail or imply necessarily that *it* exists.

Now, it is often assumed that to have intentionality is to have *content*. Mental content is otherwise described as representational/intentional or informational content and intentionality is seen as the way of bearing or carrying information. If we say what the intentional content of a state of mind is we thereby determine the conditions that must be met if this content is to be satisfied (i.e. the conditions of its truth). Thus if I believe that

"David Cameron is the British Prime Minister" my belief has a certain content thereby describing the conditions under which it is true.

Propositional attitudes are typical examples of intentional states (Figure 4.1). In the case of a propositional attitude, one expresses an attitude (a belief, hope or fear) towards a proposition. One may believe or hope or fear that *p*. The propositional content is expressed by the sentence that complements the verb. A representational state then involves a relation between a subject and a "content" (what is meant) via an attitude towards the proposition that the sentence expresses. A representational property of a representational state may thus be described as a pair composed of an attitude and a content. To say that a mental state is representational is to say that it presents the world as being a certain way. Hence representational states have *correctness conditions* partly determined by their contents. A belief, for example, is correct just in case its content is, and the proposition that gives that content is correct just in case it is true.[2]

Since a representational state consists of an attitude and a content (the intentional or representational "object"), there are two things that distinguish one intentional state from another: the attitude and the content, that is, the

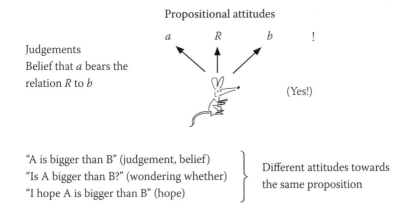

Propositional attitudes

Judgements
Belief that *a* bears the
relation *R* to *b*

(Yes!)

"A is bigger than B" (judgement, belief)
"Is A bigger than B?" (wondering whether)   } Different attitudes towards
"I hope A is bigger than B" (hope)   the same proposition

Figure 4.1 The term "propositional attitudes" refers to relational mental states that relate persons to propositions. A proposition is the factual content expressed by a declarative sentence that we take it to be expressing or affirming the way things are and is therefore capable of being true or false. In this illustration, the letters "*a*", "*b*" represent objects and "*R*" represents a relation. We can form a number of different attitudes (judgement, belief, desire, hope, fear, etc.) towards the same proposition, that is, I may judge *that a is bigger than b*, or I may hope (or fear for that matter) *that a is bigger than b*. Further, the proposition is not to be identified with the sentence; the same proposition can be expressed by different sentences: "The government has decided to hold a public inquiry into the affair" and "It was decided that the government would hold a public inquiry into the affair" (and "the snow is white" and "schnee ist weiss") would express the same proposition, or in other words, the same factual content.

intentional object.[3] But, as we said, the object is intentional, that is, the object does not necessarily have to exist. Brentano has famously argued that the distinctive feature of the mind is that it can bear relations to nonexistent objects. Asked the question "What are you thinking about?", one may answer "ghosts" or "the fifth element" or "aether". This way we can specify the content of an intentional state or its intentional object. The directedness or aboutness of the mind enables it to have intentional objects, to be related, if you will, to nonexistent objects.[4]

Generally, the notion of representation entails one thing's standing for something else (or itself in self-representation). Representing is not instantiating. Universals or objective properties (e.g. colours) are instantiated by particulars (or in the environment). In general, the mind does not instantiate the properties it represents. An object's shape, for example, is instantiated in the environment and it is represented in one's perceptual experience. For a better illustration of this point we might contrast what we might call the "representational" with the "instantiation" view of "phenomenal character". According to some representationalists (Dretske 1995; Lycan 1996; Tye 1995) the qualitative or phenomenal characters of our sensory experiences, that is, the apparent objects and properties of those experiences, are merely representational, namely they *comprise* or *contain* the content of those experiences without that content thereby being actually instantiated in the mind. Contrariwise, according to some philosophers (Chalmers 1996; Russell 1998) when I experience a red tomato, for example, the content of that experience involves the instantiation of an oval red object or the properties of this object in the mind. On this view, the object or the property of looking red is not representational. They are intrinsic properties of the mind.

It is, of course, not a straightforward matter that intentional states are physical. Admittedly, though, significant progress has been made in the project of naturalizing intentionality. There are many different attempts to provide a physicalist reduction of intentionality. Dretske (1995) and Ruth Millikan (1993), for instance, have tried to explain the intentionality of mental states in terms of their biological functions, which might in turn be given a reductive account in terms of evolutionary theory. It is expected that future work will bring us closer to a complete naturalization of the mental.

One reason for being optimistic about this is that intentionality does not seem to require consciousness; it seems wrong to say that consciousness has some primacy over intentionality. *Contra* Galen Strawson (1994, 2005), for instance, we saw in Chapter 3 that there is no reason why we should not allow that propositional attitudes such as beliefs and desires (paradigmatic intentional states) occur unconsciously. Furthermore, there are cases, such as the subliminal perception of words (Marcel 1983), where semantic information about a word (what the word means) seems to be extracted unconsciously by a subject. And considering the cases of unconscious or subliminal perception we saw earlier, it seems plain that a subject's (intentional) behaviour is being influenced by the detection of a stimulus of which the subject remains unaware. In those cases, too, it seems that the subject's behaviour is caused by an intentional state, that is, a *contentful* state, whose content is not accessed by the subject's consciousness. To admit that the content of those states can be specified in terms of what they are *about* is to admit that these states are intentional too. These considerations suggest that intentional states can occur unconsciously, or that at any rate they do not require consciousness. Thus rejecting the Cartesian picture of the primacy of consciousness over intentionality and extending the treatment of intentionality to that of consciousness, the representationalist is thereby showing that if intentionality is well understood in representational terms, then so can be the phenomena of consciousness.

4.2 REPRESENTATIONALISM, QUALIA AND PHENOMENAL EXTERNALISM

Now we can ask: what about our mental qualitative states? Are these states intentional? Are perceptual experiences and bodily sensations (being paradigmatically qualitative) representational states? We saw above that beliefs, for instance, are exemplary representational states: they are either true or false depending on whether the world is as their subjects believe it to be and false otherwise. Beliefs have accuracy conditions: they are accurate in certain circumstances and inaccurate in others. According to the contemporary representationalists, our mental qualitative states, too, including perceptual experiences and bodily sensations, are by their nature such that *they present the world as being a certain way* and therefore are assessable for accuracy.

However, it is not clear whether we should group *perceptions* and *bodily sensations* together since it looks more likely that the former but not the latter have an intentional structure (they are composed of an attitude and a content). One can *see*, for instance, *that the cat is on the mat* or *hear that dinner is ready*. But consider, for example, a feeling of elation or an experience of throbbing pain. There is something it is like for us to have these states too, but they do not seem to represent anything. Towards what are pains and itches, for example, *directed*? What are moods *about*? Both bodily sensations and moods do not seem to have an intentional object in the way perceptual experiences do, on at least the ground that although we normally distinguish between, say, a visual *experience* and *what it is an experience of*, we do not make this distinction regarding pains and moods. The latter do not seem to be about anything in the relevant sense. Consider, for instance, our use of the words "pain" and "see" in hallucinatory cases. Whereas we typically regard someone with phantom limb pain as *really* being in pain, we do not think that someone who is hallucinating an apple really sees an apple. It seems as though, in the case of pain, we focus on the *experience,* while in the case of vision we are more focused on *what it is an experience of;* as in the case of belief where we focus on *what is believed* and not on *believing,* in the case of perceptual experiences too, we seem to focus on *what is perceived.*

In a Brentanian fashion however, contemporary representationalists claim that all mental phenomena are representational, including pains, itches and emotional feelings. According to Tye (2000), for instance, pain is a representation of damage or disturbance to the body (I discuss his view in detail in §4.4). And the fact that there is something it is like for one to have a pain sensation consists in the fact that this (physical) state of affairs is re-presented in a certain way. The same holds for other qualitative properties (or qualia), such as colours, tickles and orgasms. A pain represents damage, a tickle a represents a mild disturbance, orgasm is a "sensory representation of certain physical changes in the genital region" (*ibid.:* 118), and so forth. If that is right, granted that intentional states do not require consciousness and certain mental states by virtue, say, of having the right sort of intentional content are sufficient for experience, it appears that this line of thought is very likely to provide an explanatory account of experience.

This is the other *relocationist* view of qualia that I briefly touched on in Chapter 2, that is, one of the attempts to naturalize qualia or to oppose the long-standing traditional association of their qualitative and the experiential character with the non-physical. According to this strand of representationalism, the qualitative properties inherent in our experiences are *identical* to *represented* external environmental states or features. So when one perceives a red rose, for instance, one is visually representing the actual redness of the rose. The represented redness of the rose is the actual redness of the rose itself. Thus redness is not a property of one's experience but an externally constituted property of the perceived physical object. On this view, qualia are not qualities of the experiences of, say, hearing, smelling and tasting, but rather qualities of public surfaces, sounds, odours and so on. In this sense, qualia are out there, in the external world. This view is called *phenomenal externalism.*[5]

Dretske for example, writes that "representationalism is an externalist theory of the mind. It identifies mental facts with representational facts, and though representations are in the head, the facts that make them representations – and therefore the facts that make them mental – are outside the head" (1995: 124). And Tye, in the foreword to his *Ten Problems of Consciousness,* writes that:

> not only are the phenomenal or felt aspects of our mental lives representational but also (relatedly) they are not even in the head

at all. So, neurophysiology certainly will not reveal to us what it is like to smell a skunk or to taste a fig. Look at the neurons for as long as you like, and you still will not find phenomenal conscious-ness.   (1995: xi)

The representationalist then, on facing the question "How do the wisps of protoplasm in the visual areas of the brain give rise to the redness of red?", replies that the answer is to be found not in the human nervous system but in the environment. Qualia are features of the subject's environment and the subject merely *re*presents what is presented. Avoiding the whole host of problems generated by Russellian sense data,[6] the representationalist answer is that qualia are representational contents. William Lycan writes:

> If the greenness is (indeed) not a first-order property of an imma-terial sense-datum, then of what is it a property, and/or, what kind of property is it? We must relocate it ontologically. And I maintain ... that this is a very difficult metaphysical problem ... Suppose Ludwig is seeing a real tomato in good light, and naturally it looks red to him. He is visually representing the actual redness of the tomato, and veridically so ...   (2001: 18–19)

> Of course, color realism has been a minority position in the his-tory of philosophy, so this must be counted as a liability of the Representational theory. What physical property of a lemon is it yellowness supposed to be? For the record, I buy into D. M. Armstrong's Disjunctive Realism, the view that a color is a wildly disjunctive but perfectly real physical property.   (*Ibid.*: 20)

So when one perceives a red rose, one is visually representing the actual redness of the rose. The represented redness of the rose is the actual redness of the rose itself. But what if the subject is hallucinating? Suppose that one is hallucinating a red rose and that there is actually no red rose in his visual field. In this case redness is an intentional inexistent: it is a property of the non-actual material thing (rose). The object does not exist but it is still an intentional object. If these considerations are on the right track then we learn something about the nature of qualia.[7] And, indeed, the representationalist claims to have solved the big problem of locating qualia ontologically.[8]

Tye adds:

> One's visual experience, as one views the leg, non-conceptually represents such features as color, shape, orientation of surface, presence of an edge ... If I see the moon, I am not aware of a

subjective visual field that represents the moon. I am aware of the moon and perhaps some stars located in distant regions of space before my eyes. Likewise, if I have a pain in my leg, I am not aware of an image that represents my leg. I'm aware of my leg and its condition. To suppose that it is the representation itself – the subjective visual field or the body image – of which I am really (directly) aware in these cases is like supposing that if I desire eternal life, what I really (directly) desire is the idea of eternal life. That, however, is not what I desire. The idea of eternal life I already have ... It seems to me, then, that the right thing to say is that when I attend to a pain in my finger, I am directly aware of a certain quality or qualities as instantiated in my finger. Moreover, and relatedly, the only particulars of which I am then aware are my finger and things going on in it (for example, its bleeding) ... My experience of pain is thus *transparent* to me (or so I continue to hold). When I try to focus upon it, I "see" right through it, as it were, to the entities it represents.   (2003: 282–3)

Colors, in my view, are just as perceiver-independent as shapes .... They are *real, external, objective* properties even though they are of no interest to creatures lacking our visual systems .... Indeed, on my view, colors are not presented to us in sensory experience under any mode of presentation at all. Our awareness is direct.
(*Ibid.*: 284, emphasis added)[9]

On this view, then, qualitative character is one and the same as the property of an external object (externally constituted) that appears as the content of a representational state, which, in case it meets certain specifiable conditions, brings about a certain subjective feel, that is, it is experienced.

4.3 THE ARGUMENT FROM TRANSPARENCY OF EXPERIENCE

As became apparent in the preceding Tye quote, one of the main reasons for holding the phenomenal externalist view – apart from the difficulty in locating qualitative properties in the brain or in the mind – is the *argument from the transparency of experience*.[10] This is roughly the idea that our experiences are transparent or diaphanous. However, it is not easy to find in the literature a straightforward argument from the transparency of experience to the truth of phenomenal externalism. So let us first see what the transparency thesis is commonly taken to be and I shall then attempt to sketch the transparency argument.

According to representationalists (Harman 1990; Tye 1995, 1998), we normally see through perceptual states to external objects and we do not actually notice that we are in perceptual states; the properties we are aware of in perception are attributed to the objects perceived. Visual experiences, for example, are transparent to their subjects. Tye writes:

> Suppose you are facing a white wall, on which you see a bright red disk. Suppose you are attending closely to the colour and shape of the disk as well as the background. Now turn your attention from what you see out there in the world before you to your visual experience. Focus upon *your awareness* of the disk as opposed to the *disk* of which you are aware. Do you find yourself acquainted with new qualities, qualities that are intrinsic to your visual experience in the way that redness and roundness are intrinsic to the disk? Surely the answer to this question is "No".
>
> (Tye 1998: 653)

The point is that when one turns one's attention inwards to one's experience of the certain features of the world, one is aware of the very same features. According to Tye, no new features over and above those in terms of which we characterize what it is like to have an experience are revealed. We can, of course, be aware of the fact that our mental state is representing them, but our experiences are like transparent sheets of glass and therefore we are not introspectively aware of our visual experiences any more than we are perceptually aware of transparent sheets of glass. Now, since introspection reveals no new properties at all, all experiential properties (including qualitative properties) are external:

> If we try to focus on our experiences, we "see" right through them to the world outside. By being aware of the qualities apparently possessed by surfaces, volumes, etc., we become aware that we are undergoing visual experiences. But we are not aware of the experiences themselves. (Tye 2009: 261)

And elsewhere:

> Focus your attention on a square that has been painted blue. Intuitively, you are directly aware of blueness and squareness as out there in the world away from you. Now shift your gaze inward and try to become aware of your experience itself, inside you, apart from its objects. Try to focus your attention on some intrinsic feature that distinguishes it from other experiences, something

other than what it is an experience of. The task seems impossible: one's awareness seems always to slip through the experience to blueness and squareness, as instantiated together in an external object. In turning one's mind inward to attend to the experience, one seems to end up concentrating on what is outside again, on external features or properties.   (Tye 1995: 30)

As it turns out, the main idea of the transparency thesis is that we have direct access (we are directly aware) of properties of external objects. We are not directly aware of any experiential properties. We are directly aware of intentional features of our experience, namely the objects and properties our experience is *about* and these are properties of external objects, not properties of our experiences. Introspection reveals no new properties (i.e. intrinsic to our experiences) in addition to those possessed by external objects. Thus because introspection reveals no qualities or properties of experience of which we are directly aware, we have direct access to (we are directly aware of) only the external objects and properties that are represented in perceptual experience.

The transparency thesis, then, is the claim that when one has a conscious experience one is only conscious or directly aware of what the experience is an experience of; one is directly aware of only the external objects and properties that are represented in perception. We may stipulate, then, that the first premise of the transparency argument is this (P1): we are directly aware of only the properties of external objects and these properties are represented in perceptual experience. The conclusion of this argument is that the qualitative properties in virtue of which there is something that it is like to be in a perceptual state (qualia) are properties of external objects that are represented in perceptual experience (C). What is the missing premise? A plausible premise is that we are directly aware of the qualitative properties in virtue of which there is something that it is like to be in a perceptual state.[11] Here is one way, then, to formulate the argument from transparency of experience (ATE1):

> P1. We are directly aware of only the properties of external objects (that are represented) in perceptual experience.
> P2. We are directly aware of the qualitative properties in virtue of which there is something that it is like to be in a perceptual state.
> Conclusion. The qualitative properties we are directly aware of are not properties of perceptual states but rather are properties of external objects that are represented in perceptual experience.

Now, *prima facie* there is a problem with P1, namely with the transparency thesis.[12] The problem involves cases of illusion and hallucination. It may be objected that what someone is directly aware of are not the properties of external objects in front of him; he may be unaware of what an experience is actually of (owing to illusion, hallucination, etc.). Relatedly, it is not at all clear that qualitative content does not outstrip representational content, or that introspection does not reveal any qualitative properties that are intrinsic to our experiences. Indeed, Tye's claim that we cannot be directly aware of qualities of experience seems to be false (see Block 2003). Tim Crane gives an illustrative example. He writes:

> I remove my glasses and things seem blurry. Introspecting this experience, blurriness does certainly seem to be instantiated somewhere ... blurriness does seem to be a property of some kind, which does seem to be instantiated somewhere. Unlike when things are seen *as* blurry, it doesn't seem to be instantiated by the objects of experience. So what is wrong with saying that it is instantiated (in some way) in the experience itself? Moreover, since I do not have to make myself aware of blurriness by first making myself aware of other things – the awareness of blurriness comes along all together with the awareness of everything else – introspection of seeing blurrily does seem to reveal a case of being "directly aware of qualities of experience" in an uncontroversial sense of that phrase.   (2006b: 130–31)

It does seem, then, that there are cases that show that we can be directly aware of qualities of experience.[13] But I am not going to pursue this objection any further. I shall argue that the transparency thesis should not be accepted on different grounds. Let us, then, remain neutral as to how damaging the objections from illusion or hallucination to the transparency thesis are and restrict its application to only veridical perceptions. Let us also allow Tye to maintain that introspection cannot reveal any new properties in addition to or beyond the way something looks (sounds, etc.). Hence, P1 now becomes: we are directly aware of only the properties of external objects in *veridical perception*. Here is a way to reformulate the argument from transparency of experience (ATE2):

P3. We are directly aware of only the properties of external objects (that are represented) in veridical perception.

P4. We are directly aware of the qualitative properties in virtue of which there is something that it is like to be in a veridical perceptual state.

Conclusion 2. The qualitative properties we are directly aware of are properties of external objects that are represented in veridical perception.

The problem with ATE2 is that P3 clearly begs the question. What exactly is the evidence of introspection to tell us that introspectible properties (qualitative properties) are nothing over and above the (externally constituted) properties of external objects? Does introspection tell us that an object's looking bluish to us is one and the same thing as the surface property of blue that the object instantiates? No. Introspection tells us that perceptual experience only *appears* transparent or diaphanous. This means that objects do not necessarily have the properties we seem to perceive them to have *independently of our experience of them.* Thus, it does not follow that the external world has exactly those properties. What does follow is that the external world *as we experience it* has those properties. There is nothing in perception or introspection *per se* to show that what we are directly aware of are properties of the external world. I cannot rule out (via introspection) the view that an object's looking bluish to me is a quality of my experience that I have in addition to my awareness of blueness as being the surface property of blue that the object instantiates. In other words, I might be aware of the blueness of external objects in virtue of being aware of that property of my experience.

If we are to think thus (and I do not see any reason that we should not), then it seems that the only way that the representationalist can sustain the purported claim of the transparency thesis is to add to the evidence from introspection the *assumption* that there holds an identity relation between qualitative character and external properties or content. But, of course, in this case, one does not use the transparency thesis to establish the identity relation; one uses identity to establish the transparency thesis. The transparency thesis presupposes the very identity that it purports to establish. Hence the transparency thesis is not independent evidence for identity and one cannot use the transparency thesis to establish identity.[14]

But even if we do not succeed in relocating qualia, that is, identifying them with externally constituted properties of objects (Lycan 1996, 2001, 2006; Tye 2000) or with neurophysiological states in the brain (Block & Stalnaker 1999), we do not need to eliminate them in order to naturalize them. We saw in the previous chapters that there is good reason to think that mental qualitative properties (or qualia) are not essentially conscious. That is, even if one is in a mental state with one of these properties, it does not follow that one is in a conscious state. Since qualia can occur unconsciously, they are not essentially the objects of consciousness (and in that sense non-physical). Consciousness in the relevant sense is a matter of there being something it is like for the subject to be in a mental state. The mental qualitative states that we are not aware of (perceptual or sensory states) are not conscious: if one is not in any way aware of a mental state or that one is in that state then there is nothing it is like for one to be in it. If one is not aware of what it is like then there is nothing it is like for one. This leads us to divide philosophical labour and to characterize qualia and consciousness (i.e. what it is like to have them) independently of each other and employ different explanatory accounts for them. And if qualia can occur unconsciously then they can be defined in objective terms, for example, in terms of functional roles. Thus, to conclude, if qualia are not essentially conscious then they are open to third-person examination; they will be amenable to scientific investigation. This way we solve two problems at once: first we diminish the intuitive force of spectrum inversion scenarios (since functional roles cannot be inverted), and second we naturalize qualia, avoiding the dilemma of relocation or elimination.

I said that, according to representationalists, that there is something it is like for one to have a pain sensation, for instance, consists in the fact that this (physical) state of affairs is re-presented in a *certain way*. On this view, qualitative character is one and the same as the property of an external object (externally constituted) that appears as the content of a representational state that, in case it meets *certain specifiable conditions*, brings about a certain subjective feel, that is, it is experienced. Since all qualitative mental states that meet these conditions are – invariably – conscious, the occurrence of a *certain kind* of first-order mental qualitative states is *sufficient* for experience. On this view, then, there is still a necessary tie between mental qualitative properties and experience. Thus we have not yet shown that all manner of first-order mental states (qualitative or not) can occur unconsciously. To this, I shall now turn.

4.4 EXPERIENCES *À LA* TYE

For a start, note again the distinction between first-order representationalism (FOR) and higher-order representationalism (HOR). According to FOR, some representational states (first-order), that meet certain conditions, are by their nature sufficient to give rise to experience (e.g. Dretske 1995; Tye 1995). A higher-order state about a given first-order state is not required for that given state to be a conscious state. On the other hand, HOR theories of consciousness hold that first-order representation does not suffice to account for the distinction between conscious and unconscious states. According to HOR, a state is a conscious state just in case it is the object of a higher-order mental state. The latter is a state that represents or is about the lower – first-order – state.

Dretske's (1993, 2006) and Tye's (1995, 2000) FOR accounts have been very influential, so I shall take them as exemplary. In this section, I shall look at Tye's representationalist account of experience and in the next discuss Dretske's account. In the last section of this chapter, we shall see that first-order or dispositionalist views face serious difficulties. In the meantime, I shall show that there other, additional worries for such accounts.

Let us start with Tye's view. Tye's principal aim is to defend what he calls "strong representationalism"; namely, the view that phenomenal character is one and the same as representational content (that meets certain specifiable conditions). We must note that the representationalist usage of the term "phenomenal character" is the same as the Block–Chalmers usage, that is, it means conscious qualitative character. The representationalist claim, then, is that the conscious qualitative character of our perceptual and sensory states is identical with their representational contents. The idea is that the occurrence of a certain *kind* of representational content is sufficient for experience. According to Tye, first-order experiences are first-order representational states. These first-order states are experiences by virtue of having the right sort of content. As Tye has repeatedly said, *all consciousness is a matter of representational content* (1995, 2000). The occurrence, then, of the right sort of representational content is, according to Tye, sufficient for experience.

Yet, according to Tye, we can distinguish between conscious and unconscious states in terms of certain properties of their contents. Tye does not deny that there can be unconscious representational states. Although he holds that all consciousness is a matter of representational content, it appears that unconscious perception is not a problem for his account. It would initially seem that there is a problem for FOR views such as Tye's since it might be objected that there are unconscious representational states such as unconscious beliefs or unconscious perception. So it would appear that there is no entailment here: representational (qualitative) content does not entail conscious qualitative character. And if you are a first-order strong representationalist like Tye then your account certainly requires an entailment, because identities require entailments. "Being H_2O", for instance, entails "being water". Since identities require entailments of this sort, and representational content does not entail conscious qualitative character, Tye's strong representationalism is false, that is, representational content cannot be identical to conscious qualitative character. In other words, since mental states can represent unconsciously, representational contents are not (by themselves) sufficient for consciousness. Something else appears to be required for conscious representation (no matter if the representation is qualitative or not).

According to Tye, however, this argument poses no threat to FOR: Unconscious representational content has not yet met certain specifiable conditions, it is not *PANIC*. This is an acronym for the kind of content that

Tye has in mind when he says that all consciousness is a matter of representational content. Tye's particular version of representationalism holds that our conscious states consist in those mental representations that are poised (to influence our beliefs and desires), and have abstract, non-conceptual (roughly, as opposed to propositional content of beliefs), intentional content. Conscious qualitative character is one and the same as poised, abstract, non-conceptual, intentional content (or PANIC).

Tye claims that all consciousness is a matter of representational content, but he appeals both to *functional role* and to a *certain type* of *content* in order to account for the difference between conscious and unconscious representation or between the conscious way and the unconscious way of representing a certain content. Crucially, it is not really the occurrence of the type of content that Tye postulates as sufficient for consciousness; it is the functional role or poisedness that accounts for this difference. As it turns out, "P" is the essential requirement; "P" does the trick, that is, distinguishes conscious from unconscious qualitative contents. This means that Tye's account is in essence dispositionalist and, as such, it faces all the problems that other dispositionalist accounts face, including those of Dennett (1991a), Carruthers (2000) and Dretske (2006). I shall discuss dispositionalism more thoroughly in §4.6. First, let me flesh out the claim that Tye's account is essentially dispositionalist.

Tye argues for an account according to which sensory states interact with higher-level states. A mental state is conscious just in case it bears a certain relation to conscious thoughts or beliefs. The content of the non-introspectively conscious states (or first-order experiences) must be PANIC. Now, suppose that the content of some of our first-order mental states is ANIC. If one thinks that this suffices for consciousness, then such content, namely of the kind that is representational, non-conceptual and abstract, would be sufficient for first-order experiences. But the occurrence of non-conceptual and abstract representational content is not sufficient for experience (even if it is qualitative). Tye admits unconscious representations. He also uses "representational" interchangeably with "intentional". By "abstract" content, Tye means content into which no particular concrete objects or surfaces enter. This is required by cases such as illusion and hallucination and in general to account for cases of misperception. But it is clear that the content of propositional attitudes is intentional. Further, propositions are abstract entities. Can our propositional attitudes, such as desires and beliefs, occur unconsciously? According to most philosophers they can. As I have argued, we have no reason to adhere to the Cartesian picture of the mind. The mind is not transparent to itself and there is good reason to believe that even qualitative states can occur unconsciously.

How about the requirement that conscious content be non-conceptual? Is it the case that our propositional attitudes can occur unconsciously because they are conceptual? This is absurd. And I do not think that Tye really means that conscious content must necessarily be non-conceptual. We should take Tye to mean that one can find oneself in a conscious mental state even if one does not possess the relevant concept. It is worth noting, however, that unless non-conceptuality is a necessary condition for experience, ANIC cannot be sufficient for experience. But if we take Tye to mean that the content must necessarily be non-conceptual, he must provide an answer to this simple, but serious objection. Tye draws a sharp distinction between perceptual experiences and conceptual states in the sense that the former are non-conceptual.[15] But it is not clear why non-conceptuality would be required in order for a state to be such that there is something it is like for one to be in it. Suppose that a subject came to possess the concept of "yellow16", for instance. Would that mean that the subject loses the ability to experience that shade to which the concept applies? No, it is clear that the subject would still have the ability to experience that shade. Moreover, if we agree with Tye that the content of our qualitative states is non-conceptual then we have good reason to believe that they can occur unconsciously. Recall my discussion of concept learning that leads one to experience new sensory qualities (Chapter 3). The more we enrich our conceptual repertoire, the more sensory qualities we are able to experience.

I think we should take Tye to mean that that the experience of seeing yellow16 is not itself an employment of that concept. The vehicle of the representation that is the seeing of yellow16 is not that concept. And we should take him to mean that, of course, if the subject has the concept then they can go on to make the judgement: that was yellow16. The N of ANIC is Tye's attempt to distinguish mental qualitative from mental non-qualitative states (propositional attitudes). The former do not employ concepts, but the latter do. Tye may then agree that one's coming to possess the concept yellow16 does not preclude one from consciously seeing yellow16. Thus since non-conceptuality is not necessary for experience, the occurrence of an ANIC is not sufficient for experience. Something must be added on to turn those unconscious qualitative contents into conscious qualitative contents.

So here we are. Recall that one of the conditions of the PANIC theory is that the content of mental states be poised. By this Tye means that these contents "must be ready and in position to make a direct impact on the belief/desire system. To say that the contents stand ready in this way is not to say that they always do have such an impact" (1995: 138).[16] Elsewhere he writes about what it is for a content to be poised: "This condition is essentially a functional role one. The key idea is that experiences and feelings, *qua* bearers of phenomenal character, play a certain distinctive functional role" (2000: 62). According to Tye, then, poised content is the sort of content that is available to make a direct difference to beliefs and desires, and it seems that poisedness essentially accounts for the distinction between conscious and unconscious qualitative content. Clearly abstractness and intentionality cannot account for this distinction since they are present in our propositional attitudes (nor can non-conceptuality).

Tye, like Block, holds that there is room to draw a distinction between phenomenal and non-phenomenal consciousness: only phenomenal consciousness results in subjective *feels*. Tye argues that the distinction between qualitative and non-qualitative conscious states lies in the further distinction between the *two different kinds of contents* these states have. Conscious qualitative states or perceptual experiences, according to Tye, represent "external environmental states or features". Now if the contents of perceptual experiences – namely, what these states represent – are external environmental states or features, it would seem that subjective feels (what-it-is-likeness or experience) directly depend on those features (qualitative properties). It would seem that what is suggested regarding the distinction between conscious and unconscious qualitative states is that it is in virtue of certain environmental features (representational content) that some qualitative states are conscious (have what-it-is-likeness or subjective feels). But since it appears that all environmental features can be represented consciously or unconsciously, the task of identifying those features that are required for conscious qualitative states is far from possible.[17] Thus, we are left with poisedness, that is, a dispositional role defined functionally. Before I get on to dispositionalism, I would like to raise another worry for Tye's account.

Tye claims that "honey bees like fish, *are* phenomenally conscious: *there is something it is like for them* ... And the evidence strongly suggests that some insects are phenomenally conscious" (2000: 180, emphasis added). This claim, besides being deeply counter-intuitive, is at odds with Tye's initial characterization of what it takes for a mental state to be such that there is something it is like for one to be in it. Tye postulates that some first-order states are experiences (or non-introspectively conscious) by virtue of being disposed to become introspectively conscious. So Tye must then grant honeybees and insects the ability to introspect their first-order states, that is to say, the ability to have conscious beliefs. Tye, however, denies that he is committed to this view. He replies as follows:

> I have sketched demands that phenomenally conscious states be *introspectible*. I am certainly not committed to the view that honeybees can introspect any of the contents of their minds ... [honeybees] in the higher-order sense are unconscious automata – they have no cognitive awareness of their sensory states. They do not bring their own *experiences* under concepts.
>
> (2000: 181–2)

A couple of paragraphs below Tye suddenly transforms into a HOR theorist. He writes

> [I]f indeed simple creatures like honey bees are inherently blind to their inner states, then, although they are the subjects of phenomenal consciousness, they never *suffer*. *Suffering requires the cognitive awareness of pain. The person who has had a bad headache and who is distracted for a moment or two does not suffer at that time. The headache continues to exist ... but there is no cognitive awareness of pain and hence no suffering. In the phenomenal sense however, the pain still exists even though its subject is briefly blind to it.* (*Ibid.*: 182, emphasis added)[18]

Tye concludes by saying that "whether or not simple creatures feel pain, without the power to introspect they do not suffer" (*ibid.*).

Tye's account is problematic on at least two grounds. First, he says that although honeybees have *feels*, they do not have any *sufferings*. To be able to suffer or to experience the hurtfulness of pain, says Tye, requires a higher-order state: the cognitive awareness of pain. It is here that Tye's view sounds exactly like a HOR view. Clearly, suffering or the hurtfulness of pain cannot occur unconsciously. At any rate, it sounds counter-intuitive to suggest that it can. What I have been suggesting is that together with all first-order qualitative states, pains can occur unconsciously, not that the hurtfulness of pain or suffering can occur unconsciously. The *experience* of pain cannot occur unconsciously. And this is precisely for the reason that Tye mentions: the first-order pain state becomes the target of cognitive awareness (a higher-order state) and this, in turn, explains why there is something it is like for one to be in that – pain – state. Is there still something it is like for one to have a headache if one does not suffer at that time or if the pain does not hurt (if we are "blind", as Tye puts it, to the pain)? Does one still *experience* the pain? It is far more plausible to say that although mental qualitative states can occur unconsciously, they are not experienced. As Rosenthal puts it, the person who has a headache and is distracted does not suffer at that time; the headache continues to exist, but there is nothing it is like for one to have that headache (whenever one is "blind to it").

Second, notice that Tye is committed to the view that honeybees and some insects have conscious mental lives; that is, he does not merely say that honeybees and insects have unconscious mental qualitative states, he says that these are *experiences*. Bees, according to Tye, are "subjects of phenomenal consciousness". As he explicitly says, "there is something it is like for them" to be in those states. At the same time he says that blindsighted states are not phenomenally conscious because they are not poised to directly influence rational control of behaviour and action; they are, so to speak, ANIC. As he puts it, "blindsight subjects do not believe their guesses" (2000: 63). This is a fair point about which I shall have to say more in the coming chapters. But do honeybees and insects believe their "guesses"? Tye says that "they do not bring their own experiences under concepts"; "they are inherently blind to their inner states" (*ibid*.: 182). What is the difference, then, between these two kinds of states?

I think that Tye cannot maintain both claims: namely, that blindsighted states are not phenomenally conscious (for the reason that, as he also says, they are blind) and that the honeybees' states (or the insects' states for that matter) are (since P is missing from these states too). In both cases, we are dealing with states of an organism that *cannot* become introspectively conscious (as Tye says, the subjects are blind to their inner states). Both states are ANIC, not PANIC, and, according to Tye, ANIC is not sufficient for experience, or "phenomenal consciousness" in his terminology. ANIC is the vehicle for pain but it is not sufficient for having a pain experience. Since Tye holds that blindsighted states are not experiences and honeybees' states are (the former are not *because* P is missing and the latter are *despite* missing P) his position is inconsistent.

But what reason could we possibly have to credit honeybees and insects with conscious mental lives? Why not say that caterpillars, too, find themselves in mental states or that there is something it is like for them to undergo some of their mental states? Tye says that there is no reason to believe that caterpillars move purposefully: "they do not believe that the light is strongest at the tops of the trees ... they do not want to get to the strongest light ... nothing in any of their behaviour seems to require the admission that they have any wants or beliefs" (2000: 174). So, Tye concludes, intuitively, there is no reason to attribute phenomenal consciousness to a caterpillar. On the other hand, according to Tye, there is good reason to attribute phenomenal consciousness to honeybees and to some insects. He uses metaphorical language to convince the reader that honeybees move purposefully. He writes:

> scouts fly out from the hive each spring in search of a cavity suitable for a new hive ... upon returning, they dance to show bees in the hive what they have discovered ... scouts back from their trips attend to the dances of other scouts and then go out again to visit the different cavities. (*Ibid*.: 178)

He points out however, that some of this is pre-programmed in that bees choose neither to dance nor how to navigate. But, says Tye, bees "learn and use facts about their environments as they go along ... honey bees are very good at detecting and remembering odors ... they can identify one odor among 700 others" (*ibid*.: 178–9).

I would be happy to endorse Tye's line of argument to the effect that mental qualitative properties (and not experiences) can occur in bee states. However, metaphorical language aside (since one could equally use the same language to describe the behaviour of caterpillars), Tye does not offer us any good reason to think that, *contra* our intuitions, bees and insects undergo conscious qualitative states in that even notebooks and laptops seem to have a similar learning capacity.[19] And, plausibly enough, laptops do not have subjective feels or experiences. However, there does seem to be a difference between laptops and honeybees in that we would hesitate to attribute sensory states to laptops. At the same time, it is indeed deeply counter-intuitive to attribute subjective feels and experiences to simple creatures, such as honeybees and insects. One cannot fail to notice in Tye's claims the importance of cognitive abilities, such as conscious thoughts and beliefs for experience. Granted the importance of such abilities and since Tye cannot hold both that ANIC is and is not sufficient for what-it-is-likeness, the only position available to him is to say that if an organism lacks such cognitive or introspective abilities it cannot enjoy any experiences (or phenomenally conscious states, as Tye calls them); otherwise he is committed to an incoherent position. But this is a high price to pay: consider for how many non-human primates (even human babies) we would hesitate to say that they possess the capacity to introspect or to reflect on their mental lives and the mental lives of others.[20]

4.5 EXPERIENCES *À LA* DRETSKE

In this section, I shall try first to sharpen the dispositionalist view by contrasting it with Block's view. I shall then look at Dretske's dispositionalist view of experience. Recall that, according to FOR, there is a dispositional role that distinguishes conscious from non-conscious states. However, FOR theorists typically maintain also that A-consciousness (recall Block's dispositional notion of accessibility) *is* required for first-order experiences (Dennett 1991a; Carruthers 2000; Tye 2000). They hold, against Block, that accessibility to the content of the first-order experiences is required in order for those states to be able to become introspectively conscious. Indeed, blindsight and visual extinction cases show us precisely that lack of access to the content of certain mental states results in there being nothing it is like for one to be in them.[21] Tye notes (*contra* Block) that the case of blindsight shows that even when mental states have the right sort of intentional qualitative content, there is nothing it is like for one to be in those states. The content of blindsight states *cannot* become introspectively conscious because the blindsight subject is *not able* to form or express an assertoric attitude towards the content of those states. Merely guessing or wishing that one is in a certain state cannot make that state conscious. As Tye put it, blindsighted subjects cannot believe their guesses.

Recall that, according to FOR, non-introspectively conscious states are experiences because they are disposed to cause conscious beliefs (higher-order states), and blindsight states, although they somehow bear a relation to higher-order states, cannot become introspectively conscious, that is, they cannot cause or bring about conscious beliefs (similarly with other cases presented in Chapter 3, such as visual-form agnosia and visual extinction). Blindsight states, then, are *not disposed* to become introspectively conscious and hence, according to FOR, they are not experiences.

Most FOR theorists agree. Tye, for instance, writes that "the function (or a function) of phenomenal consciousness [experience] is simply to enable creatures to use information represented in their brains in the guidance of rational action (as contrasted with guessing behaviour)" (2004: 122).[22] Thus, according to FOR, although no access is required for experience (in the sense that the first-order state be the actual target of an occurrent thought or perception) accessibility is required (Block's dispositional notion of A-consciousness). Although blindsight patients store visual information (qualitative), they seem to lack a certain kind of direct introspective access to the visual modality or to the corresponding sensory content. And since, plausibly enough, there is nothing it is like for them to undergo this state (they do not experience the stored visual information), it appears that if a mental state lacks a pattern of access to its (qualitative) content it cannot be an experience.

Here is what Lawrence Weiskrantz, who discovered the phenomenon, says about the blindsight patients: "All these subjects lack the ability to think about or to image the objects that they can respond to in another mode, or to inter-relate them in space and in time; and this deficiency can be crippling" (1991: 8). Since there is a complete lack of access to the sensory content of those states, any sensory-modality-based mode of mental representation is absent in those cases. The content of blindsight states, then, cannot become introspectively conscious; hence, there is nothing it is like for one to be in those states because one cannot even become conscious of being in them. On this – FOR – account, it appears that there is room to maintain a distinction between conscious and unconscious representational qualitative states. Conscious qualitative states are the sort of mental states that *are able* to become introspectively conscious. Thus blindsight and similar cases do not pose any problem for this FOR variant.[23]

Suppose now that the blindsight patient, when he finds himself disposed to "guess" that there is a cross on the paper, for example, comes to believe that he sees the cross because the experimenter whom he trusts tells him so. Or, becoming knowledgeable about his condition, he forms a theory that when he is inclined to "guess" cross it is because he is seeing a cross. Still, the advent of such higher-order beliefs does not cure his blindsight; he still does not *consciously see* the cross. Nor would it be enough for the higher-order belief to come to him spontaneously and without rational ground. For it is conceivable that some future investigator might be able to induce that higher-order belief in our patient spontaneously and without it having a rational ground from the patient's viewpoint, just by pressing a button that activates directly appropriate nodes in his belief area, so our patient as well as having the inclination to plump for the answer "cross" also finds himself believing that he sees it, as he did formerly on the experimenter's testimony, while yet not consciously seeing it.

I suggest that what we need to constitute *consciously seeing* the cross, what we need for there to be something that it is like for him to be seeing the cross, is for him to believe that he is seeing the cross *on the rational ground of his being visually aware of the cross.* I propose that, for a subject to be *consciously seeing* a red patch, for example, is for the subject to see a red patch and believe that he sees a red patch, and the first cognitive state is, from the subject's point of view, the immediate rational ground of the second: the subject does not from her point of view have the belief ground-lessly, nor have it on such indirect grounds as the testimony of the experimenter or the subject's own internalized theory of blindsight whereby his inclination to guess becomes for him a symptom of his seeing. I shall have more to say about this proposal in Chapter 6, where I will formulate a HOR account of experience.

That all said, let me now turn to Dretske's account of experience. Dretske (1969) draws a distinction between epistemic and non-epistemic visual perception. Imagine, for instance, that you are driving too fast to identify some obstacle lying in your path, but you adeptly manage to avoid hitting it. Unless you saw it you would have hit it. Since you did not hit you saw it. But you failed to identify or notice it. (Cases of peripheral vision provide similar examples). This perception, according to Dretske, is non-epistemic. Non-epistemic perceptions occur in those cases where one *sees* something but fails to *notice* or *identify* it. According to Dretske, in this example, we have a case of an unconscious perception that is, however, in *some sense* conscious. Although non-epistemic perceptions occur unconsciously, they are, according to Dretske (1993, 2006) conscious, in that although there is something it is like to be in them, one is not aware *that* one is in those states.[24]

According to Dretske, first-order states are first-order experiences not by virtue of one's being aware of them: one is only aware *of* the thing one sees, not *that* one sees it. On this view, one's being "aware of" the thing is treated as synonymous to one's seeing the thing without thereby being in any way aware *that* one sees it. Awareness *that* is judgement-like, epistemic, propositional and conceptual. Hence experience on this account does not necessarily come in propositional form.

Of course, from being aware *of* the thing, it does not follow that one is aware *that* one sees it or that there is something it is like *for one* to see it. And Dretske is certainly right to say that sensory states can occur unconsciously. But the real issue here is whether these states are somehow conscious: in other words, whether there is still something it is like for one to be in those states. Dretske writes: "what we are asking, remember, is not merely whether *perception* of something can occur without awareness of it, but whether *conscious* perception can occur alongside a belief that one is aware of nothing" (2006: 159). Dretske's answer is yes. It is worth mentioning that a few years ago, Dennett regarded Dretske's non-epistemic seeing as being not interestingly different from what happens on the inert wall of an unoccupied camera obscura. "You need to add some sort of uptake", Dennett suggested, to justify saying that details are "in consciousness" in the sense that they are not also on the wall in the camera obscura.

> Do you still think that there is a theoretically interesting sense of non-epistemic seeing that does not just collapse into something like "ephemeral cortical activity was the result of retinas being irradiated by light from" (or alternatively into something that is a non-ordinary variety of epistemic seeing after all)?
>
> (Dretske *et al.* 1998)

Dretske replied:

> Dan thinks the richness of the outside world, in all its ravishing detail, does not enter our experience of that world. I think a lot of this richness, this detail, does enter our experience. Not all of it, of course, but more of it than we notice or respond to ... I am, in fact, quite happy with the results of these experiments. They show what I would expect to be shown, what I take to be obvious – viz., that a lot of what we see we don't notice. They do not show that we do not see things unless we notice them. They only show that if we see these things in a non-epistemic way (as I claim we probably do), epistemic seeing does not always accompany non-epistemic seeing. (*Ibid.*)

It is certainly true that a lot of what we see we do not notice. Behavioural evidence suggests that subjects can see something without being aware that they saw it. But why agree with Dretske that these subjects are *consciously seeing* something with the belief that they are aware of nothing? As Dennett puts it: "what is it like, for instance, to use information about the optic flow of shapes in peripheral vision to adjust the length of your stride as you walk across rough terrain? The answer is, it isn't like anything. You can't pay attention to this process even if you try" (2001: 17).

Most importantly, Dretske faces the threat of contradiction. In claiming that conscious perception of something can occur without awareness of it, Dretske seems to claim in effect that we can have an unconscious perception that is nonetheless conscious. *Prima facie*, this is a contradiction: "unconscious" entails "not conscious", so seemingly he is saying that a subject can be both conscious and not conscious. This is impossible. And this is not the only place or case where Dretske claims of some perception that it is both unconscious and conscious. One other such case is Armstrong's (1968) absent-minded driver. According to Armstrong, when one is driving very long distances in monotonous conditions one can come to at some point and realize that one has driven many miles without being conscious of the driving. Let us construct a case such as the following. Suppose that while driving I pass something (I did not notice what it was and therefore I have no conscious beliefs about it) and after a while a friend asks "Have you seen *that*?" I reply, "You mean the red thing with the kind of rectangular shape standing nearby the fence?" Clearly, in this case, my (first-order) perceptual state was able to be introspectively conscious, in other words, it was poised to cause a conscious assertoric attitude. The question now is this: was my unconscious perceptual state, being evidently a state disposed to become introspectively conscious since I eventually became (introspectively) conscious of it, experiential? Is my unconscious state of perceiving the red pillar box a non-introspectively conscious state?

Here is what Dretske writes about such cases: "The only sense in which it is unconscious [mental state] is that the person whose state it is is not conscious of having it. But from this it does not follow that the state itself is unconscious" (1993: 271). *Prima facie*, this does not seem to make much sense. Dretske says that the person is not conscious, "but it doesn't follow that the state itself is unconscious". This is a very peculiar claim. We have taken talk of mental states being conscious as a mere shorthand for the person being conscious, where what they are conscious of is somehow specified by the mental state. It simply does not make sense to attribute consciousness literally to a mental state itself.

Thus we need to look for a charitable reading of Dretske. Dretske says that *the only sense* in which it is unconscious is that the person whose state it is is not conscious of having it. I think that Dretske's account is to be understood analogously to a disjunctive theory of perception.[25] That is to say, there is not one state, consciousness, which can be achieved by two different routes (sense perception and propositional attitudes). As disjunctivists deny a common factor to seeing and hallucinating, so Dretske is denying that there is a common factor to consciousness-of and consciousness-that (hence the hyphens). They are not two different kinds of the same state, consciousness. Now there is no contradiction: the person is conscious-of and not conscious-that. However, as I have been arguing, I believe that consciousness is a single state, which can be subdivided by its objects. And this has two advantages over Dretske's position: one theoretical and the other empirical.

To see more clearly what these advantages are, we need to compare three cases: the case of blindsight, the case of the inattentive driver and, say, the case of a fully attentive birdwatcher. First, the blindsight case. In my view, the blindsighted subject is not conscious of the letter "A", say. In Dretske's view, the blindsighted subject is not conscious-of and not conscious-that. How about the inattentive driver? It is true that the driver sees the road; otherwise, as Armstrong wrote, he would end up in a ditch. But to establish the further claim that these states are unconscious *experiences* something more is needed. From merely saying that the driver still sees the road it does not follow that the visual qualitative properties involved are conscious. What follows, at most, is that visual qualitative properties such that there is nothing it is like for one to have them can occur in unconscious states, not that the driver experiences those properties.[26] In my view, such cases of shift of attention suggest that there are sensory states that are conscious only some of the time. In the case of the inattentive driver, I think, it is plausible to suggest that although he saw the red pillar box, he was not conscious of (seeing) it. By contrast, according to Dretske, although the driver was not conscious-that, since Dretske is a dispositionalist and the person could have been made so conscious by prompting, the driver was conscious-of.[27] Lastly, let us appeal to the case of an attentive birdwatcher. In my view, the birdwatcher is conscious both of, say, the robin in the bush and that there is a robin in the bush. According to Dretske's account, the birdwatcher is both conscious-of and conscious-that (in this respect, this is unlike a disjunctive theory of perception, where a perceiver cannot be in both states at once).

Now, in order for Dretske to be consistent, he has had to say that conscious-of and conscious-that are different states. But he also wants to say that there is a dispositional link between them: being conscious-of disposes one to be conscious-that. Is this an *a priori* claim of a conceptual link? Well, for one thing they are different states; there seems to be no *a priori* reason why the one should dispose its host to enjoy the other. Is it an empirical claim? There is no empirical evidence for the dispositional link in the case of the absent-minded driver. Dretske has *assumed* that the driver was conscious-of because he can be prompted to become conscious-that. There is no direct empirical evidence that the driver actually was conscious-of at the time, nor that it is this that disposes him to become conscious-that later. In contrast, a higher-order account has no need to postulate this ungrounded link between two such distinct states. It turns out, then, that Dretske's account is disadvantageous on both theoretical and empirical grounds.

Summing up then, we saw that both Tye's and Dretske's accounts of experience are first-order in the sense that they hold that first-order states are experienced by virtue of a certain kind of *dispositional role* these states have. The occurrence of a distinct (higher-order) state is not required. In the previous chapters, we saw that according to both Block and Chalmers, mental qualitative properties are essentially conscious and therefore their occurrence is sufficient for experience. Similarly, although FOR accounts can maintain a distinction between conscious and unconscious states, a certain kind of representational (qualitative) content is sufficient for experience. In this respect, FOR accounts are subject to similar objections. Further, we saw that there are additional difficulties for Dretske's and Tye's accounts. In the concluding section of this chapter, I shall present two arguments against dispositionalist accounts of consciousness in general, which strongly suggest that such accounts are inadequate to account for the phenomenon of experience.

4.6 DENNETT'S BETSY, FREDDIE AND A NEURAL MEDDLER

In this section, I shall conclude my discussion on first-order theories. I shall present two thought experiments that, I believe, put all dispositionalist accounts in a very difficult position. We shall see that no such difficulty arises for actualist – as opposed to dispositionalist – HOR accounts. Now, on the face of it, dispositionalist accounts face the rather intuitive objection that dispositional thoughts, or dispositional states in general, are merely dispositions for these states to occur and it is hard to see how mere dispositions – as opposed to occurrent thoughts, for example – can make our mental states conscious. Although this is a fair point to make, Carruthers for instance, disagrees. He claims that "what makes an occurrent thought ... to be conscious ... is that *it is made available* to further thought through the operation of a regular feed-back loop whose function is to make such thoughts available to yet further thoughts" (1996: 195, emphasis added). These thoughts, then, are conscious not by virtue of the occurrence of a higher-order thought (HOT) but because they are available as the contents of HOTs.[28] In a similar spirit, Tye (2000) and Dretske (2006) suggest that non-introspectively conscious states are conscious because of a certain kind of a dispositional role these states have. On all these accounts, mental states are conscious simply because they can produce conscious HOTs. They do not have to produce these thoughts.

The first objection comes from William Seager (n.d.) and serves well to illustrate a general advantage of actualist over dispositionalist accounts, fleshing out the intuition that dispositional thoughts or dispositional states in general are merely dispositions for these states to occur and mere dispositions cannot make our mental states conscious. Seager objects as follows. Suppose that we have some kind of machine, call it a "neural meddler", that interfered with the cognitive mechanisms that normally permit the first-order state to cause that HOT which makes the former conscious. We would thus have a "consciousness inhibitor". Now, consider a neural meddler that blocks the disposition to cause or bring about higher-order states only for those states and for those time periods when the first-order states would not, in fact, cause a HOT. As Seager points out, such a meddler would be extremely difficult to produce in practice but, of course, the practical difficulty of developing such a meddler is irrelevant to the point at issue. Seager writes:

> Let us take two people, one with a neural meddler attached to his or her brain and one without, but who otherwise begin in identical neurological states (and in identical environments). Both of these people will have an identical history of higher-order thoughts, since the meddler will never prevent a lower [first] order state that actually was going to produce a higher order thought from causing that thought. They will also have identical histories of lower [first] order mental states, for the meddler has no effect on these. Yet they will be markedly different in their states of consciousness, for the unfortunate person with the meddler will lack an entire set of conscious states enjoyed by the other – namely those that as a matter of fact do not produce any higher order thoughts (but – in the unmeddled brain – could). (n.d.: 8)

This is a necessary consequence of dispositionalism as it is intended to allow that states are conscious by virtue of being able or available to produce HOTs (or higher-order states in general). It is easy to see now why this consequence of dispositionalism is highly implausible. As Seager succinctly puts it:

> There is absolutely no difference in the behaviour of our two individuals and no difference in their history of mental states. There is nothing to mark the difference between the two of them except an *entirely inert* meddler. The meddler never has to actually function to produce this drastic alteration in consciousness. That is, two brains identical in their neural states and their dynamics will differ in consciousness solely because one has an *inert* piece of machinery within it! (*Ibid.*: 9)

Of course, since according to an actualist HOR theory, we become conscious of our first-order mental states by virtue of an occurrent higher-order state about them, no such difficulty is presented for such a theory.[29]

The problem becomes more apparent if we further imagine that the meddler is oscillating between being "off" (incapable of functioning) and being "on" (capable of functioning even though it never will). As Seager puts it, in this case:

> here will be a corresponding oscillation in consciousness (more conscious states when the meddler is disabled, fewer when it is enabled) which would presumably be very striking but in fact would … seemingly be completely unreportable by the subject despite being a huge difference in phenomenological experience.
>
> (*Ibid.*: 9)

These consequences of dispositionalism are indeed difficult to swallow. But there is a more serious objection to dispositionalist accounts of experience and to this objection I shall now turn.

We saw previously that according to FOR, non-introspectively conscious states are experiential by virtue of being disposed to bring about introspective conscious states such as conscious thoughts and beliefs. So if we take the case where someone's current visual experience is directed at an environmental setting featuring a blue armchair right in front of him, he will become conscious of this aspect of the setting just in case this aspect is suitably poised to bring about a belief to the effect that there is a blue armchair right in front of him. The portion of the content of the sensory state (the aspects of the environmental setting), then, that is suitably poised to bring about the higher-order state is experiential. In other words, according to FOR, there is something it is like for one to be in this first-order sensory state because the state is disposed to bring about introspectively conscious states.

Hence, we can say that according to FOR, there is something it is like (E_1) for one to be in a first-order sensory state with content C_1 because it is suitably poised to bring about a conscious belief *that* C_1. Similarly, it would be like something (else) (E_2) for one to be in a first-order sensory state with content C_2 because it would be suitably poised to bring about a conscious belief *that* C_2 (of course, C_2 may be suitably poised to bring about the belief *that not-* C_1). Since C_1 and C_2 are different, E_1 and E_2 would be different experiences. Recall that according to most dispositionalists, first-order states are experienced by virtue of their content (which meets certain specifiable conditions). This content is in a position to make a (direct) impact on the belief–desire system (Tye 1995, 2000). To generalize the point, representational contents that meet certain conditions are disposed to bring about higher-order states and therefore they are experiential. Thus, as it turns out, experiences on the FOR account are to be individuated in terms of their contents,[30] that is, in terms of the representational or functional role they play in human cognitive economy.

Now, there are two sources of trouble. First, most philosophers agree on what we might call the *singularity of conscious content*. This means, roughly, that we experience only one unified and cohesive (in the sense of consistent and organized) environmental setting at once.[31] Second, and in relation to the first point, since experiences are characterized by the role they play in the belief–desire system, a single experiential content cannot play two contradictory roles simultaneously. That is, it is hard to see how a certain content can become experiential by *being disposed to bring* about the belief *that p* and *bring about* the belief *that not-p* at once. I shall attempt to illustrate these points by means of the following two examples.

Suppose that at a certain time *t*, Freddie was looking for a cufflink in one of his drawers. Freddie failed to find the cufflink, yet he discovers afterwards that it had been in full view in the very drawer in which he had been looking. If Freddie was aware *that* he was perceiving the object, he would have found it. But Freddie did not find it. It seems, then, reasonable to suppose that this perception was not noticed by him. From this, two things follow: either there was no (unconscious) perception of the object at all,[32] or there was one but Freddie was not aware of it at the time. But if the perception did occur, then Freddie would have been in a perceptual state the representation of which necessarily includes the cufflink.

Let us suppose that there is evidence that the second hypothesis is correct. Freddie's behaviour suggests that he actually saw the cufflink but in fact he had failed to find it (Freddie does not want to go to the party for some reason and he managed to self-deceive). If, say, Freddie's behaviour suggests that he actually saw the cufflink, which, in turn, suggests that he experienced it according to dispositionalists, then how can we consistently say that at *t* Freddie was in a perceptual state with a single representation in which he both *experienced and did not experience* (since he failed to notice it or find it) the cufflink? Can Freddie at *t* have two contradictory experiences of the same representation (a conscious and an unconscious one)? In other words, can Freddie at the same time, both experience and not experience the cufflink: can he have two contradictory experiences simultaneously? And what kind of content exactly does Freddie experience at *t*?[33] Note that this has nothing to do with whether or not Freddie remembers his experience. If you ask Freddie two minutes after his search he will say that he did not find what he was looking for.

There are two options for the dispositionalist, neither of which is satisfactory. Recall the point about the unity of experience: the content of experience is singular; we experience only one unified and cohesive content at once. In our case, however, things are different. A single representational content is disposed to bring about the belief *that p* and brings about the belief *that not-p* simultaneously. This is because at *t*, Freddie believes *that not-p* while his behaviour suggests that he unconsciously believes *that p*. Now, the dispositionalist must *either* (i) say that perceptions that go unnoticed (non-epistemic) are such that there is something it is like *for one* to be in them, *or* (ii) opt for Block's notion of "experience", which leaves subjectivity or "for oneness" out. If (i), then the subject finds himself having contradictory experiences: since experience is defined as a mental state such that there is something it is like *for one* to be in it, then there is something it is like for Freddie to experience *p* and *not-p* simultaneously. But what would it be like for Freddie to be in this state? If (ii), then the position fails to account for "experience" in the Nagelian sense. As we saw in Chapter 3, Block's sense of "what-it-is-likeness" is not what Nagel was getting at. Nagel's notion leaves no logical room for a sense of "what-it-is-likeness" that does have to do with the mind but leaves subjectivity out. Although we can form this concept of "what-it-is-likeness" (since there is nothing such that it is not like something – there is something it is like to be a leaf on a tree, namely, being a leaf on a tree) it is a concept that has universal extension. And an experience is a mental state such that there is something it is like *for one* to undergo it.

It should now be clear why neither option will do. If the notion of the unconscious "what-it-is-likeness" is not the Nagelian one (and, as I have argued, it cannot be) then dispositionalism fails to account for experience since first-order states of the required kind are such that there is nothing it is like *for one* to undergo them. If the dispositionalist holds that first-order states of the required kind are such that they possess "what-it-is-likeness" in the Nagelian sense, then Freddie finds himself to have contradictory experiences. In this case, it is open for the dispositionalist to say that there may be something it is like for one to be in a mental state that *S* and not-*S* simultaneously. However, neither option is good enough: the first leaves Nagelian subjectivity out, and the second, bearing in mind the point about the unity of experience, implies that Freddie finds himself having an inconsistent experience; indeed, something very odd is happening to him.[34] But we can avoid this dilemma by simply saying that for some reason although Freddie saw the cufflink he failed to notice it and therefore did not experience the presence of the cufflink. Why should we think that our lives may include such contradictory experiences or why should we think that there is any interesting theoretical sense in freely using the term "experience" whenever a perceptual discrimination occurs? Indeed, if all seeing (both conscious and unconscious) is experiencing, we cannot even begin to ask what it is for a particular state to be experiential or wonder why some seeing is.

A case not unrelated is the following. Restaurants, classrooms and lecture halls typically have chairs (and tables) that usually have the same colour, same shape, size and so on. It is normally the case that when you walk into a restaurant you do not need to closely observe all the chairs in the room to form a belief about them; it normally takes you only a few seconds to have a look around the room and have a belief to the effect that the place looks like this or like that. This includes the paintings on the walls, the shape and colour of the chairs, the tables and so on. Now, a few weeks ago, a friend invited me to dine with him in a restaurant I have never been to before. When I walked into the room (at time t_1) I saw, among other things, the brownish colour of the chairs and tables as well as the nice decoration on the walls. We sat at a table in the corner and started looking at the menu. My friend had not told me anything about that place, except that it was one of his favourite restaurants. When I suddenly looked at the cutlery on the table, I discovered to my surprise that mine were different from his; both the shapes and sizes were different. It was clear that they belonged to a different set. When I made him aware of this he just pointed to the chairs and said, "See they're all different. And look at the tables they're all different too." Apparently this was one of the things for which this restaurant had a reputation (as well as good food): everything was one of a kind. But at t_1 I experienced being in a place in which all the chairs had the same shape, colour and so on. I did not notice their exact shape and colour. Plausibly, then, it can be said that having a belief about those chairs "smoothed them out" so I experienced them as ultimately homogeneous. And whereas it may be also (plausibly) urged that I did see the actual shapes of the chairs and tables when I walked into the room, what determined my experience, what it was like for me to be in the particular mental state, was my judgement *that* the chairs were all the same, not the fact that I was probably aware *of* their actual shapes and sizes.[35]

Another example comes from Dennett. In order to distinguish between perception and awareness, Dennett appeals to the once very popular children's game Hunt the Thimble. The point of this game is to become aware of what you are already perceiving and the whole fun of it is when someone that tries to find it is counted on to "look right at the thimble several times without actually seeing it" (1991a: 334). In these moments, everyone else can see the thimble, which is right in front of Betsy's nose, but she just cannot find it. Before Betsy becomes aware of the thimble, says Dennett, even if some representational state in Betsy's brain *includes the thimble*, "no perceptual state is about the thimble yet". This is followed by a distinction that Dennett draws between being in the foreground of experience and being in the background of experience. Dennett further distinguishes these two senses of experience from the sense in which a mental qualitative property is merely in the background of the perceptible environment (without being an experience). Thus a distinction between *experiences* and *perceptions* (non-experiences) does feature on Dennett's account.

However, according to him, awareness *that* or *of* a mental state is not required for the state to count as an experience. Dennett distinguishes between the two varieties of experience as follows. In order for a perception to be in the foreground of one's experience there must be some special relationship of intentionality or aboutness between it and some other of my mental states. According to Dennett, what must happen is for Betsy to:

> "zero in on" the thimble, to separate it as a "figure" from "ground" and identify it ... The thimble will finally be "in her conscious experience" – and now that she is conscious of it, she will be able at least to raise her hand in triumph ... Such feedback-guided, error-corrected, gain-adjusted, purposeful links are the prerequisite for the sort of acquaintance that deserves the name – that can then serve as a hinge for policy, for instance. Once I have seen something in this strong sense, I can "do something about it" or do something *because* I saw it or *as soon as* I saw it.
>
> (*Ibid.*: 335)

The kinds of intentional relationships required for Dennett, then, are these feedback-guided, error-corrected, gain-adjusted (purposeful) links. Betsy's achievement of concentrating on the thimble is an achievement, says Dennett, that calls for more than a single "momentary informational transaction". Betsy manages to experience the thimble in this sense because this visual process leads to other processes in the brain that in turn make possible a HOT about it. As Dennett says, I can then "do something about it".

Dennett says that both foreground and background experiences are characterized by reportability: if something is in the background of experience then it is reportable whereas when something gets into the forefront it is "getting in a position where it can be reported on" (*ibid.*: 336). Dennett's account then falls in the category of dispositionalist accounts, according to which a mental state is conscious or experiential in so far as it is disposed to bring about or make HOTs possible.[36]

According to Dennett, the items or objects in the background of the experiences can be singled out at any moment by any of those intentional acts mentioned in the paragraph above. What gives them this disposition is past experience. Dennett invites us to consider the case of a professional piano tuner. Piano tuners are trained in such a way that they "come to be able to isolate, in their auditory experience, the interference beats, and to notice how the patterns of beats shift in response to their turning of the tuning 'hammer' on the peg" (*ibid.*: 337). As is widely believed, training and the learning of new concepts can alter our experiences. The case just presented is exemplary. As a result of the tuners' training says Dennett, their experience has changed.

Next, Dennett invites the reader to imagine that one of these professional tuners is absorbed in conversation with someone in a room where an out-of-tune piano is playing. Although the tuner may not be aware of the fact that the piano is out of tune because he is not really listening to it, if the piano stopped playing he would notice it. What is more, according to Dennett, he would even be able to tell you which notes exactly were out of tune and this is because even though he was not conscious of the experience, the experience of listening to the piano was there all right. How else, asks Dennett, could we possibly characterize this state as experiential other than ascribing to it a dispositional role that enables it to bring about higher-order states? On this account, a higher-order state (awareness) is not required for experience. Items in the background of the experience are experiential because they are disposed to be singled out by an intentional act, which in turn brings about higher-order states about them, and therefore these items become the objects of awareness. Awareness in this sense can shift from one object or content to another, but this object or content is itself experienced because of its disposition to bring about those states of awareness.

Recall Freddie's case. Freddie was looking for a cufflink but could not find it. Here we have a similar case. Betsy is allegedly conscious of, or experiences, the thimble both before and after she discovers it. Again this leads one to think that at a certain time t, Betsy both experiences and does not experience the thimble. Now, this again leaves one wondering what exactly is the content of the total, unified experiential state that Betsy finds herself in since, as Dennett explicitly says, *the representation of the unconscious experience may include the thimble.* How can Betsy, at t, have two contradictory experiences of the same representation (a conscious and an unconscious one) and what is it like for Betsy to be in that mental state? In other words, what is it like for Betsy to both experience and not experience the thimble at once? Does she still experience a unified and consistent content? It is hard to see how that might be so. It is most natural to say that the representation includes the thimble but it is *merely* disposed to bring about the belief that p, that is, it is only a disposition for a thought to occur which has not as yet occurred, and therefore there is only one experiential state that Betsy finds herself in at t, namely the one she is aware of, the content of which does not include the thimble.

Things are worse for Dennett, since on his account there are two layers of unconscious experiences: background and foreground experiences, which are both characterized by the notion of reportability. If something is in the background of the experience, says Dennett, it is reportable, whereas something getting into the forefront of consciousness is "getting in a position where it can be reported on". While Dennett never really explains what the difference is between "reportable" and "getting in a position where it can be reported on", it is clear that both are dispositional notions. So if an experience is characterized by its dispositional role we can easily construct another thought experiment to make a case where a background experience is disposed to bring about the belief that *p* and a foreground experience is disposed to bring about the belief that *not-p*. A single representation could then be disposed to bring about the belief that *p* and *not-p* simultaneously (we may say that *p* is reportable and *not-p* is in a position where it can be reported on). So, again, one would find oneself having contradictory experiences, even before conscious beliefs get in play. So it appears that Dennett has two options: *either* the Dennettian background and foreground "experiences" do not refer to the Nagelian notion of what-it-is-likeness, or Betsy finds herself to have contradictory experiences. Neither option is satisfactory: an explanatory account of experience must both (a) encompass the idea that experience is consistent and (b) satisfy Nagel's criterion. Dennett is forced to abandon one of these requirements. Thus an actualist higher-order account is much more satisfactory since on such an account we can consistently uphold both (a) and (b).

Relatedly, according to Dennett, there is nothing in our experiences about which we are fallible. We cannot have such mental phenomena and not know or believe that we have them. That is to say, there is no existence of our experiences independently of what we believe about them.

> You seem to think there's a difference between thinking (judging, deciding, being of the heartfelt opinion that) something seems pink to you and something *really seeming* pink to you. But there is no difference. There is no such phenomenon as really seeming – over and above the phenomenon of judging in one way or another that something is the case. (1991a: 364)

This is one of the central tenets of Dennett's "heterophenomenology" (roughly, the idea that third-person examination of people's reports about what they believe their experiences to have been provides a fully adequate basis on which to explain experience). But now suppose that Betsy believes at a certain time that she did not see the thimble (or that her experience did not include the thimble). Why still think that she nevertheless experienced it (in the sense that there is something it is like for her to see it)? Since, according to Dennett, our experiences cannot exist independently of what we believe about them and Betsy may be staring at the thing but firmly denying that she sees it, then, plausibly, Betsy does not experience it. Betsy sees it, but not consciously so: there is nothing it is like for her to see it.

5. EXPERIENCE AND THE EXPLANATORY GAP

5.1 THE STORY SO FAR

We saw in previous chapters that we have good reason to think that qualitative properties can occur unconsciously. There is a large amount of evidence that shows that our unconscious states have effects on behaviour and other mental states independently of whether or not the state is conscious. In Chapter 4, we saw that dispositionalist accounts are highly implausible; first-order states do not become conscious in virtue of a dispositional role these states may have. First-order mental states can occur unconsciously independently of whether they are qualitative or of whether they are suitably disposed or poised to bring about certain higher-order cognitive states. Thus, not only can non-qualitative mental states, such as our beliefs and desires, occur unconsciously, but all manner of perceptions and sensations can exist in both conscious and unconscious modes.

We saw previously that both qualitative and non-qualitative conscious states are experiences in the sense that there is something it is like for one to be in them. Hence, since all manner of qualitative states and properties are not essentially conscious, we have good reason to believe that the same *fundamental kind* of experience is involved in both qualitative and non-qualitative conscious states. And since the occurrence of such properties is neither necessary nor sufficient for experience, we do not experience our mental states in virtue of the occurrence of such properties. What makes certain mental states such that there is something it is like for one to be in them has nothing to do with whether or not a certain mental state is qualitative. Experience, then, must be specified independently of any qualitative properties and therefore it is explanatorily irrelevant to any qualitative properties.[1]

Our considerations suggest that a mental state is conscious by virtue of the occurrence of a distinct higher-order state about it, not simply because it is disposed to cause such a higher-order state. One cannot experience being in a particular mental state if one is not in any way aware of being in that state. Conscious states are states that we are aware of. Awareness in the relevant sense is a form of knowledge: being aware of our own mental state involves knowing that we have it. On this view, a theory of what it is to be aware of is kept distinct from a theory of what the objects of this awareness are. We are thus led to a division of labour, and to characterizing qualitative properties and experience independently of each other and employing different explanatory accounts for them. This division is the key to many difficult problems in contemporary philosophy of mind, including the notorious explanatory gap. My main aim for the rest of the book is to show that a higher-order thought (HOT) view of experience, properly construed, can soften the hard problem of consciousness and help us solve the explanatory gap problem.

In this chapter, I shall first explain the problem of the explanatory gap and then present the kind of explanation that is required to close it. We shall see that this neo-Cartesian challenge is indeed a very serious challenge to all physicalist and non-physicalist accounts of experience. It will become apparent that an appeal to neuroscience is the wrong level of explanation and that non-reductive and non-physicalist accounts fall short of providing the required explanation. But there is an alternative. We must look for an explanation at the cognitive level.

5.2 THE EXPLANATORY GAP

Contemporary neuroscience is teaching us that all the diverse experiences or mental phenomena that we typically associate with consciousness correlate with particular patterns of brain activity. All experimental data point to the fact that all these experiences are a product of brain activity and that with no brain there are no such experiences. However, although we know that consciousness arises from a physical basis, we do not have a good explanation of why and how it so arises. Pain experiences, for instance, correlate with C-fibre firing, but even if we know that the feeling of pain correlates with C-fibre stimulation and that, say, the existence of such pain states is contingent on the occurrence of such a neural event, we still want to know why it does not correlate with a neural state of another kind or why it is pain rather than the feeling of euphoria or an itch that correlates with that particular kind of neural state. This leads us to the more general question of why it is that there holds such a correlation *at all.* Trying to answer such questions raises the problem of the *explanatory gap* (Chalmers 1996; Levine 2001).

The most influential notion of explanation in the philosophy of science is the notion of *contrastive explanation*, according to which an explanation should progress by answering contrastive questions of this type: why *A*, rather than B? Broadly, a contrastive explanation (Lewis 1986; Lipton 1993; Baars 1997) is explanation of P relative to a class of contrasting alternatives. It explains why-P rather than relevant alternatives to P, that is, why P rather than Q or R or S or T? For example, why is it that water boils at 212°F rather than 100°F or 150°F or 1000°F at sea level? (There is a need for an explanation here, since it is conceivable that things could have been different than they are.) Chemistry has discovered that the liquid we call "water" is made up of molecules that are themselves made up of atoms of hydrogen and oxygen. When the kinetic energy increases sufficiently, the hydrogen bonds of H_2O help form an open lattice with a density less than that of liquid water, and other liquids do not have these bonds. Notice that this explanation has to do with the *constitution* of water. We know *a posteriori* that "water is H_2O". Because we know this (necessary) truth about water we can infer that if a certain liquid had exactly the same constitution then it would boil at 212°F at sea level and it would expand when freezing. In other words, we can *predict* that a liquid with the same constitution would behave accordingly. The higher-order properties of this liquid can be *deduced* from its constituents. In this case, we establish a *conceptual* connection. After all physical facts are filled in, the explanatory gap disappears.

But this situation is quite unlike the case of experience. Take the case of a pain experience (E_1) and of an experience of another kind, say an experience of an itch (E_2). It makes sense to ask why C-fibre stimulation brings about E_1 rather than E_2 since it could have been that C-fibre stimulation correlates with E_2 and not with E_1. Unlike the case of water, in this case even if all neurophysiological facts are filled in we are not making any progress. It is still coherent to conceive of a situation where C-fibre stimulation brings about E_2 rather than E_1. Whereas it is incoherent to conceive of a situation where the "boiling process" of H_2O mentioned above takes place at 212°F at sea level yet water at the same conditions freezes instead of boiling, it is not incoherent to conceive of a situation where C-fibre stimulation brings about E_2 rather than E_1. Citing more facts about the constitution of neural states will not help and an appeal to the qualitative difference between a pain and an itch is no good either. Since it seems that that is all we have and we do not have a clue about where else to look for an answer, there is a wide-open explanatory gap. People were not in a position to answer the question about water 500 years ago, say, but at least they roughly knew where to look for an answer.

It is true that some patterns of neural activity result in experience and other patterns do not. Identifying those patterns is an important and difficult task. Francis Crick and Christof Koch (1990), for instance, have argued that the neural basis of a visual experience with a particular qualitative property is cortico-thalamic oscillation of a certain frequency.[2] However, no relevant progress has been made in adding another neurophysiological fact or correlation to the sum of our knowledge: since experience cannot be deduced from facts about neurons, another such fact cannot fill in the explanatory gap. And further advances in knowledge of neurophysiological structure cannot provide corresponding advances in explanatory force. As Levine puts it, when we identify a certain type of experience with some type of neural state "it still seems quite intelligible to wonder how it could be true, or what explains it, even after the relevant physical and functional facts are filled in" (2001: 81–2).

It might seem that prior to the "Why A *rather than* B?" question is the question "Why A *at all*?", and we have agreed with Chalmers that the hard problem of consciousness is why there is experience *at all*. In other words, it might be objected that from our inability to answer questions such as "Why is it that a pain experience rather than an experience of a different type occurs?" it does not follow that we are not able to answer the question "Why is there any experience *at all*?" But questions such as "Why is there a pain experience *at all*?" or "Why is there experience *at all*?" are intrinsically related to contrastive questions of the kind "Why *A* rather than *B*?" Consider the case of water again. It could have been that water does not boil at 212°F at sea level. But it is not. The explanation of why water boils instead of freezing at this temperature has to do with the very constitution of water. We know, for instance, that when the kinetic energy increases sufficiently the hydrogen bonds of H_2O help form an open lattice with a density less than that of liquid water. This shows that when we are able to answer the "why boiling rather than freezing" question we are in a position to answer the "why boiling at all" question – Why does water boil rather than not boil *at all*? – because this phenomenon simply *consists in* the aforementioned process that takes place at 212°F at sea level if the liquid in question is H_2O.

Similarly, if we are not in a position to answer the "why a pain experience rather than itch experience" question, we are not in a position to answer the "why there is a pain experience *at all*" question. Indeed, although some observed physical–mental correlation gives some justice to our belief that a pain experience must occur rather than an itch experience, it is still conceivable (in the sense that it does not yield a contradictory representation or self-contradictory description) that it could have been otherwise. We want to know why it is pain rather than the feeling of anxiety or an itch that correlates with that particular kind of neural state. And appealing to the correlations themselves, or citing facts about the constitution of our neurophysiological states, cannot provide the required explanation. No matter how well informed neuroscientifically an answer may be, it would still be conceivable that a neural type of another kind correlates with pain or that C-fibre stimulation may occur without being accompanied by any pain experience at all (think of the multiple realizability objection and Kripke's argument from

§1.3). Thus it does make sense to ask "Why a pain experience rather than no pain experience at all?" And since we are not in a position to answer this question, there is an explanatory gap; namely, we do not know why there is experience *at all*.

5.3 REDUCTION AND REDUCTIVE EXPLANATION

How can we close the gap? It appears that there are two ways: *reduction* and *reductive explanation*. We can try to *reduce* the pain experience to, say, a certain kind of neurophysiological process in the brain. We could argue, for instance, that the pain experience state just is the particular type of neurophysiological state. In this sense, the statement "a pain experience is a particular type of a neural state" or "a pain experience is C-fibre stimulation" would have the same status as the statement "water is H_2O". And ontologically a pain experience would be nothing but a particular type of a neurophysiological state. On the other hand, we can attempt to *reductively explain* the pain experience in terms of, say, a pattern of neural activity. Chalmers provides a good illustration of the distinction between reduction and reductive explanation:

> In a certain sense, phenomena that can be realised in many different physical substrates – learning, for example – might not be reducible in that we cannot identify learning with any specific lower-level phenomena. But this multiple realisability does not stand in the way of reductively explaining any instance of learning in terms of lower-level phenomena. (1996: 43)

According to the "multiple realizability" argument, other physical structures such as silicon painmakers could both function and feel like ordinary pain. It is plain that the physiological basis of a pain experience may differ between species. Multiple realizability, then, is a problem for reduction because a mental property, such as a pain experience, can be multiply realized and thus it cannot be identical to any *particular* brain state. Hence we cannot identify a mental state type, such as being in pain, with a physical state type, such as a specific sort of brain state. However, multiple realizability is not a problem for reductive explanation. Even if we cannot reduce a pain state to *a particular kind* of a neurophysiological state it would suffice, as in the case of learning, to explain any instance of pain in terms of "lower-level phenomena".

Reductive explanation of experience requires the derivation of experiential statements from statements about neural or physical states and processes. There are many ways that this could be accomplished.[3] We shall, however, focus on the possibility to establish *conceptual connections* between experiential properties and physical properties (functional reduction). Chalmers writes:

> What is it that allows such diverse phenomena as reproduction, learning, and heat to be reductively explained? In all these cases, the nature of the concepts required to characterise the phenomena is crucial. If someone objected to a cellular explanation of reproduction, "This explains how a cellular process can lead to the production of a complex physical entity, but it doesn't explain reproduction", we would have little patience – for that is all that "reproduction" means. In general, a reductive explanation of a phenomenon is accompanied by some rough-and-ready analysis of the phenomenon in question, whether implicit or explicit ... The point may seem trivial, but the possibility of this kind of analysis undergirds the possibility of reductive explanation in general. Without such an analysis, there would be no explanatory bridge from the lower physical facts to the phenomenon in question.
>
> (1996: 43–4)

What form does the required "conceptual analysis" take, exactly? Chalmers writes:

> For the most interesting phenomena that require explanation, including phenomena such as reproduction and learning, the relevant notions can usually be analysed functionally. The core of such notions can be characterised in terms of the performance of some function or functions (where "function" is taken causally rather than teleologically), or in terms of the capacity to perform those functions. It follows that once we have explained how those functions are performed, then we have explained the phenomenon in question. Once we have explained how an organism performs the function of producing another organism, we have explained reproduction, for all it means to reproduce is to perform that function.
>
> (*Ibid.*: 44)

An essential element of this kind of reductive explanation (or functional reduction) appears to be *a priori* reductionism or derivation. Most philosophers in the field think that a reductive explanation requires *a priori* reductionism (Chalmers 1996; Levine 2001; McGinn 2004; Kim 2005).[4] Here is a good way to illustrate what *a priori* reductionism really means. According to Chalmers and Jackson (2001), in the case of all macroscopic phenomena *M* (e.g. "This water is liquid", not implicating what-it-is-likeness or experience), there will be an *a priori* conditional of the form $(P \ \& \ T \ \& \ I) \rightarrow M$, where P is a complete description of all microphysical facts in the universe, T is a "that's all" clause intended to exclude the existence of anything not entailed by the physical facts, such as ghosts or immaterial souls (no experiential facts or mental parts that themselves essentially require consciousness are included), and I specifies indexically where I am in the world and when now is. They argue that the existence of such conditionals is required if there are to be reductive explanations of the phenomena described on the right-hand sides of those conditionals. According to them, in a reductive explanation of a phenomenon such as water or life, we find that a low-level account of the physical processes involved will in principle imply and explain truths about the macroscopic structure, dynamics, behaviour and so on. In other words, there are such conditionals for those higher-level phenomena. These phenomena can be deduced from the lower-level phenomena on the left-hand side of the conditionals.

They write:

> When a concept of some natural phenomenon supports a priori entailments from the microphysical, there is a clear sense in which the phenomenon can be reductively explained. These a priori entailments might not support a reduction of the phenomenon in question to a microphysical phenomenon (at least in some senses of this term), perhaps because such entailments are compatible with multiple realizability. But nevertheless, in showing how any instance of the phenomenon is itself implied by microphysical phenomena, we show that there is a sort of transparent epistemic connection between the microphysical and macroscopic phenomena. (2001: 348)[5]

Note that there is a difference between reductive and non-reductive explanation as the terms suggest. According to Chalmers, reductive explanation is explanation wholly in terms of simpler entities, hence its name. By "simpler entities", we mean that "the explanatory premises of a reductive explanation of a phenomenon involving property F (e.g. an explanation of why F is instantiated on this occasion) must not refer to F" (Kim 2005: 105). The reductive role in these conditionals (in the Chalmers and Jackson case) is played by the "that's all" clause. A reductive explanation of experience (supposing that that is the phenomenon on the right-hand side of the conditional) will explain it wholly on the basis of physical principles or properties that do not themselves make any appeal to experiential properties.

Now, according to Chalmers and Jackson, experience is not reductively explainable. According to them, there are no *a priori* conditionals of the form

$(P \& T \& I) \rightarrow C$ in the case of experience, because no experiential fact C can be deduced from the left-hand side of the conditional. Thus experience or what-it-is-likeness cannot be reductively explained. Contrariwise, according to them, in the case of water we know that there are such conditionals. That is, once we fix the left-hand side of the conditional by putting all microphysical facts about water, all the facts about water are determined. Once we further add information about where in the microphysically described world I am and when now is, it looks like all the facts (including all the facts about water and excluding all facts about experience) are determined. Here is how we can restate their argument:

P1. If there are to be reductive explanations of the phenomena described on the right-hand side of the conditionals it is required that there are *a priori* conditionals of the form $(P \& T \& I) \rightarrow C$

P2. There are no *a priori* conditionals of the form $(P \& T \& I) \rightarrow C$ where C describes experiential facts [phenomenal facts in Chalmers & Jackson (2001)].

Conclusion. There cannot be a reductive explanation of experience [phenomenal consciousness in Chalmers & Jackson (*ibid.*)].

Thus experience cannot be reductively explained. The left-hand side cannot be fixed by purely physical properties (explained in terms of function and structure) or mental parts that do not essentially themselves require consciousness. Hence, according to Chalmers and Jackson, experience is unlike any other problem of cognition that we face.

Now, should we take "$(P \& T \& I) \rightarrow C$" to be a *logical* truth? If that were true then if "C" is, say, "this water is liquid", the property of being liquid will be logically entailed by the micro-properties "$P \& T \& I$" if there is to be a reductive explanation of its liquidity. In the quote above, Chalmers and Jackson talk about "*a priori* entailment" but that need not be logical consequence. If C = water is liquid, and there is no mention of "is liquid" allowed in "$P \& T \& I$", then "C" will definitely not be deducible from "$P \& T \& I$".[6] But then how do "pain = C-fibre stimulation" and "water = H_2O" differ in the relevant sense? How can Chalmers and Jackson arrive at the conclusion that experience is unlike any other problem (of cognition) that we face?

We should not take Chalmers and Jackson to mean "logical truth" by "*a priori* conditional" and I will not take it that by "deduce" they mean that C is a logical consequence of $P \& T \& I$.[7] The notion of the reductive explanation in play implies that the right-hand side of the conditional *does not follow by logical inference* from the left-hand side. Take the case of the boiling of water. Appealing to physical theory, we say that the boiling of water for instance, *consists* in a certain process that takes place at 212°F at sea level if the liquid in question is H_2O. There is an *a priori* or conceptual connection established here since the kind of explanation that Chalmers and Jackson have in mind is mediated by definitions and by definitions they seem to mean analytic definitions grounded in conceptual analysis, something that can be formulated and evaluated *a priori*.[8] The example that Chalmers gives in the quote above is this:

> Reproduction = def. organism producing another organism.

In the case of the boiling of water we might – rather tentatively – suggest the following definition:

> Boiling of water = def. process that takes place at 212°F at sea level
> if the liquid in question is H_2O.

Another word for explanation is *predictability*. When we want to reductively explain *A* to *B*, we want to show how *B* facts alone will suffice for prediction of *A* facts. Thus from the process that takes place at 212°F at sea level if the liquid in question is H_2O (*D*) we can predict (or deduce) that water boils (*G*), in other words, if *D* then G. So the claim then is that, in the case of experience, we cannot establish similar *conceptual connections* between experiential properties and physical properties, or indeed any other properties at all specifiable in non-experiential terms.

However, in order to establish a *conceptual connection* between physical properties and experience, we need, at minimum, to be able to *conceive* of *all that*, that is "*P* & *T* & *I*". But notice that we need *P* to include, among the "microphysical truths", specification of all fundamental laws of nature concerning the microphysical entities, and specification of the settings of any free parameters, for example the value of the cosmological constant. That is, *P* specifies in detail all that is necessary and sufficient to determine the total physical nature and entire physical history of our actual universe.[9] Obviously we cannot even formulate *P*, nor could we grasp it if it were presented to us. Only a hypothetical Laplacian demon can grasp *P*: the conjunction of all microphysical truths about the universe, specifying the fundamental features of every microphysical entity, all fundamental laws, all free parameters. The requirement, then, is that the relevant conceptual connection cannot be established by the Laplacian demon. But what is Chalmers's and Jackson's *warrant* for this? It seems obvious to me that there is no non-question-begging warrant for this claim. The only reason humans could have for thinking thus would be a reason for already thinking that experience is non-physical.

Yet there are currently no known physical or neurophysiological facts in virtue of which we can reductively explain facts about experience. Hence one might be tempted to think that we cannot *currently* reductively explain experience or that our current situation is such that we cannot reductively explain experience; we cannot currently establish the required conceptual connection. There are two options. First, one may accept only the *epistemic implications* (McGinn 1991; Levine 2001). This may take two forms: (i) an answer is not forthcoming in the foreseeable future (Levine 2001); (ii) an answer is not forthcoming at all – we cannot reductively explain experience in principle (McGinn 2004). Both these views, however, deny that just because consciousness cannot be reductively explained, it is non-physical or that at any rate this commits us to a kind of ontological dualism. Second, one may take it a step further. That is, one can grant both its *epistemic* and *ontological implications* and argue that arguments such as the one presented above justifies a belief in ontological dualism (Chalmers 1996). I shall first discuss these two options in more detail, in a reverse order. Then, I shall propose a reductive explanation for experience along the lines of the Chalmers and Jackson suggestion.

5.4 PANPROTOPSYCHISM

It is certainly striking that one of the most prominent contemporary physicalists' latest book is entitled *Physicalism, or Something Near Enough* (Kim 2005). Kim's desperation is obvious when, in the last chapter of his book, he arrives at a position that he calls "conditional physical reductionism". He concludes that whereas intentional (mental) states such as beliefs and desires are functionally reducible (reductively explainable), what-it-is-likeness is not so reducible. What we cannot reductively explain, says Kim, are the intrinsic qualities of our sensory experiences. He writes: "intrinsic qualities of qualia are irreducible, and hence causally impotent. They stay outside the physical domain" (*ibid.*: 173). The "intrinsic properties of qualia" stay outside the physical domain, according to Kim, because we cannot *reductively explain* what-it-is-likeness (identified according to him with this intrinsic nature). Kim, however, concludes by saying that losing what-it-is-likeness is not losing much and that this is the closest we can get to physicalism. (At least he admits that experience or what-it-is-likeness is not a fiction of bad philosophy and that it should be explained and not explained away.) But as a conscious state in the most interesting sense (Nagel 1974; Block 1995; Chalmers 1996), Kim concedes that consciousness escapes physicalism.

We saw that there is currently no physical description that could bear the required conceptual relation with experience: there is currently no physical description from which we can deduce that there is something it is like for one to be in a particular mental state. It appears, then, that experience is not amenable to physical reductive explanation. According to some philosophers (Jackson 1982; Chalmers 1996; but not Levine), from the explanatory (epistemic) gap we can infer an ontological gap: if we cannot deduce Q from P then we cannot explain experience in terms of physical processes and therefore experience is not a physical process. According to Chalmers, if (P & $\neg Q$) is conceivable it is (metaphysically) possible. Since conceivability entails possibility according to Chalmers (1996), then experience does not supervene on physical facts: two possible situations can be identical with respect to their physical properties while differing in their experiential properties.[10] Nevertheless, Chalmers thinks that an explanation for experience, albeit a non-reductive one, can be given.

According to Chalmers (*ibid.*), panprotopsychism (roughly, the view that an experiential element is present in everything that exists)[11] qualia or qualitative properties are mental in the sense of being non-physical and non-physical in the sense of being essentially the objects of consciousness. In this sense, only non-physical properties can exemplify experiential properties. According to Chalmers (*ibid.*), a mental qualitative property is an experiential item and it is constituted out of the intrinsic natures of the fundamental physical entities. The intrinsic properties of the physical world include proto-experiential properties. Chalmers postulates proto-experience as a fundamental property of physics alongside mass, charge and space–time. Although it is hard for us to see how experiential or proto-experiential properties can be explained by physical theory, they are, nonetheless, part of the physical world. As Chalmers puts it, they are integrated with the physical world. And since modern physics says nothing about the intrinsic nature of physical entities and properties such as quarks and mass, respectively, Chalmers offers a (Russellian) solution, which could solve both problems at once: *the intrinsic properties of matter are proto-experiential* (proto-phenomenal properties as he calls them).[12]

Chalmers suggests that experience supervenes on some sort of functional organization of its constituents (proto-experiential) and this enables us to explain experience: by appealing, that is, to such functional organization. He employs the notion of *organizational invariance*, according to which the same functional organization determines the same phenomenal experience (as he calls it). At the same time, he admits that although there is a systematic correlation between functional organization and experience, "this is just correlation, in the sense that it would at least be logically possible to have the functional organization without consciousness; and furthermore, that explaining the functional organization doesn't explain why the system is conscious" (Chalmers 2002b).

Of course this kind of supervenience can hardly be of the required kind, since functional accounts, according to Chalmers himself, are susceptible to the explanatory gap argument: there is no *a priori* derivation from any amount of physical and functional facts, says Chalmers, since it is still conceivable that a system could have the required functional organization and not be conscious. Chalmers's non-reductive explanation amounts to no explanation at all, since functional accounts, according to Chalmers, cannot close explanatory gaps. According to his own account, it would still be conceivable that this functional organization of proto-phenomenal properties can occur without the occurrence of experience. We still need an explanation as to how a fine-grained functional organization of proto-phenomenal elements constitutes experience. Thus it seems that Chalmers merely introduces another explanatory gap since, according to him, we cannot deduce from any kind of functional organization of proto-phenomenal properties that the subject enjoys experiences. So Chalmers's non-reductive functionalism falls short of giving us the conceptual connection that is required for an explanation of experience (albeit non-reductive).[13]

Further, if it is true that both non-reductive and reductive explanatory accounts fail to explain experience in that they both fail to close an explanatory gap, why should we go for the non-reductive explanatory variant that commits us to such heavy metaphysical assumptions? According to Chalmers, for instance, experience is constituted out of the intrinsic natures of the fundamental physical entities. This is a highly speculative claim, of course, which endorses a dualistic picture of nature (since proto-experience is introduced as fundamental) and alludes to panpsychism. I think that alluding to panpsychism is too high a price to pay. For one thing, according to Chalmers's view, if information – defined in a sense in which every physical difference that makes a difference in the world is information (1996: 281) – is what gives rise to experience, then as he correctly observes, there must be experience everywhere. But this is deeply counter-intuitive, and we are given very little, if any, independent grounds to believe why it could be so (one such motivation Chalmers uses is Jackson's knowledge argument; see §1.3).

Instead of falling into the trap of wondering whether there are conscious systems to be found in rocks, the starting point must be why or how certain physical systems give rise to experience and other systems that lack the required structure do not. It seems both metaphysically and scientifically outrageous to suppose (having no physiological and behavioural signs) that rocks actually have feelings, emotions and thoughts that they happen not to be able to communicate. This brings to mind the case of the Presocratic philosopher Anaxagoras. Anaxagoras, sometime around 450 BCE, posed the following question: how could hair come from what is not hair or flesh from what is not flesh? He suggested that the philosopher Empedocles was wrong in positing in the "original mixture" *only* the so-called "four elements". Nothing comes into being from not-being. As opposed to Empedocles, in his list of the ingredients of which everything consists, there were not solely four elements. To his mind, Empedocles had not gone far enough. According to Anaxagoras, in everything there is a portion of everything. Since nothing comes into being from non-being, hair must come from what *is* hair. And since in everything there is a portion of everything there must be little hair somewhere inside the head from which could come hair! One cannot fail to notice the resemblance that the "in everything there is everything" story bears to Chalmers's story, that is, the striking resemblance that "little hair" bears to "little experience" or proto-experience. It appears that there are no independent grounds on which one could add experience to mass, charge and space–time.

There is another interesting analogy that Dennett (1996) draws in this connection. According to him, some things are just plain cute and other things are not cute at all. Because it is hard to explain or describe why, we had better postulate proto-*cuteness* as a fundamental property of physics alongside mass, charge and space–time. These analogies, I think, drive the point home. As I said previously, these are some of the symptoms of the conjunction of two highly misleading assumptions; namely, that our mental qualitative properties are invariably conscious and that the right way to close the explanatory gap is to appeal to neuroscience. Even if we abandon the first assumption, an appeal to neuroscience to close the gap faces insurmountable difficulties, I have argued.

5.5 MCGINN'S MYSTERIANISM AND SEARLE'S BIOLOGICAL EMERGENTISM

Our inability to come up with a reductive explanation of experience led McGinn (1989a, 1991, 2004) to take the step from "we cannot currently reductively explain experience" to "we cannot explain it *in principle*". McGinn thinks that there is an explanatory property to fill the explanatory gap. However, owing to our *cognitive closure*, the property is "noumenal" for us.[14] According to the so-called "mysterian", the explanation of the hard problem of consciousness is beyond our powers of understanding: even if alien beings were to explain to us how the gap closes, we would not understand. As he says, we can identify P – the property that can fix the left-hand side of the required conditional – neither by direct investigation (introspection) nor by empirical study of the brain. Since these two ways are blocked we cannot identify P. Hence we are cognitively closed to *how* it is that brains generate experience. This problem is not solvable, but an unsolvable mystery.

However, cognitive closure with respect to this explanatory property does not imply irrealism about *P*. It is simply that *P* is inaccessible to us by perception and introspection yet it may be grounded in physical properties. Therefore, whereas the problem can be solved in principle (some possible beings might be able to solve it), owing to our limitations of understanding it will remain forever closed to us. In a pessimistic spirit similar to Kim's, the mysterian points out that since the problem has stubbornly resisted our best efforts, it is probably time to admit that we cannot resolve it or that at any rate an answer is not forthcoming.

According to Searle however, McGinn's pessimism is not only premature (as Chalmers would say) but wrongheaded. In *The Rediscovery of the Mind* (1992), he argues that McGinn takes Nagel's argument a step further (since he thinks that the mystery cannot be solved *by us in principle*) on the basis of mistaken Cartesian assumptions. Searle argues that the very terminology of the field is one of the main sources of trouble. According to Searle, experience is not some kind of "stuff", but a property of the brain, in the sense that liquidity is a feature of water, and it is not known by introspection in a way analogous to the way objects in the world are known by perception. Experience is not an "object" for inner inspection, says Searle. According to him, experience is like solidity or liquidity. Searle thinks that McGinn's mistake crucially is that he thinks that there is a "link" between experience and some property of the brain. According to Searle, as there is no "link" between liquidity and H_2O molecules, there is equally no "link" between experience and the brain. McGinn (1991) explicitly denies this analogy. He says that the dependence of liquidity on the properties of molecules is exactly *unlike* the dependence of experience on the brain, since in the former case the relation is *spatial* in character and we can also employ the idea of spatial composition.

McGinn thinks that there is a link between experience and the brain; the to-us-unknowable *P* will reveal the hidden structure of consciousness, the *missing link* between the brain and experience. In *The Problem of Consciousness* (1991), McGinn argues that neural phenomena are spatial but experience is *prima facie* non-spatial. Echoing the alleged Wittgensteinian repudiation of a spatial model of the mind, he states:

> Perceptual geometry gets no purchase on them [conscious states].
> And this is not just a contingent fact of the mind ... We have no
> conception of what it would even *be* to perceive them as spatial
> entities. God may see the elementary particles as arrayed in space,
> but even He does not perceive our conscious states as spatially
> defined – no more than He sees numbers as spatially defined. It is
> not that experiences have location, shape and dimensionality for

eyes that are sharper than ours. Since they are non-spatial they
are in principle unperceivable.   (1995: 221)

On McGinn's assumption that there is a link between them, it appears very difficult to explain how the former give rise to the latter. Experience considered thus cannot be linked to the brain in virtue of spatial properties of the brain. How can something spatial be causally related to something non-spatial? McGinn suggests that there must be some kind of property P that can explain the mystery. It is just that, owing to our cognitive closure, we cannot know what P is.

Searle denies this conception of experience. As we have seen, on his account there is no link between experience and the brain. And experience is spatial; it is located in the brain.[15] According to him, whereas one cannot say that H_2O gives rise to water or that it is the correlate of water, one *can* say that what gives rise to a certain property of water (e.g. liquidity) is the configuration and causal relations, and so on, of H_2O molecules, or that the properties – energy levels – of the molecules give rise to liquidity. Here no explanatory property P is needed to reveal any link because there does not appear to be any causal link. And liquidity is not a kind of "stuff". Searle thinks that the same considerations apply to experience. The brain, in the same sense, gives rise to experience, which is like the emergent property, liquidity, to which H_2O gives rise, not like H_2O. Moreover, the properties of liquidity cannot be reduced to something like the properties of the molecules, and liquidity is causally efficacious. Supposing that Searle is right that there is no link between experience and the brain. Can this analogy help us to explain experience?

As far as we know, it appears that experience is far from being analogous to properties such as solidity and digestion. For one thing, unlike solidity and liquidity, the causal efficacy of experience appears mysterious. Although we can explain in purely physical terms exactly how solidity and, say, digestion are causally efficacious, causal efficacy of experience poses serious difficulties (recall that Kim, for instance, argued that it is epiphenomenal). For another, Searle in his supervenience/emergentist/biological account appears confused. On the one hand, he claims that experience is a biological phenomenon like digestion. On the other, he says that if one is tempted to functionalism, as he puts it, one does not need refutation but help: the mind is left out. I suppose no one (including Searle) holds that when digestion or liquidity is described in functional terms the phenomenon is left out. But if experience is like digestion, why is it left out when it is described in functional terms?

Searle says that neurophysiological processes give rise to mental phenomena, but he says they do not – and, cannot – *constitute* mental phenomena.

Mental phenomena can be explained by neurophysiological structures and processes, he thinks, but specific mental phenomena cannot be reduced to neurophysiological processes. But then experience is quite *un*like liquidity or solidity. When all physical facts are filled in there is nothing left over to explain in the case of liquidity or solidity. There is no outstanding explanatory gap. Searle is right to say that the solidity of an object can be explained by the behaviour of the molecules and that this does not show that solidity is nothing but the sum of the properties of the molecules or that there is no difference between solidity and liquidity. Both these higher-order properties can be predicted by the properties of elementary particles. But just because they can be explained in terms of some lower-level physical properties it does not mean that they are one and the same as the sum of these properties. (This is another illustration of the difference between reduction and reductive explanation.) However, Searle fails to see that liquidity or solidity can be predicted from the properties of elementary particles, whereas experience cannot be predicted from the properties of neurons. Whereas one can come up with an *a priori* conditional in the case of solidity and liquidity by appealing to physical properties alone, one cannot come up with a conditional in the case of experience by appealing to any number of properties of neurons. What is more, Searle gives us no reason to believe that *experience* is indeed spatial or that it is indeed somehow related to the brain in virtue of spatial properties of the brain. So it appears that Searle is merely reiterating the problem: experience is somehow brought about by neurophysiological processes in the brain but we do not know how.[16]

Summing up our discussion so far, we saw that we cannot reduce experience to brain states and, further that we cannot give a reductive explanation of experience (in physical or neuroscientific terms). Further, non-reductive explanatory strategies such as Chalmers's fail since they too cannot provide the required explanation (let alone the heavy metaphysical assumptions that they carry with them). Is the mysterian right then? Is it true that we cannot, even in principle, close the explanatory gap? It very much looks as if the discussion should be focused on whether a reductive explanation is forthcoming in the near future, or not coming at all. According to McGinn, it is not coming at all.

5.6 WHAT ARE WE TO DO?

Carruthers (2000) argues that there are at least two major faults in the mysterian account. I disagree with the first. Without getting into too much detail, Carruthers suggests (in accordance with Owen Flanagan [1992]), that there may be no specifically cognitive constraints on knowledge acquisition.

This view strikes me as highly implausible. For one thing, assuming that the story about the origin and the evolution of the species is for the most part true, if one admits that certain cognitive constraints would not allow, say, *Australopithecus afarensis* to understand certain truths of quantum mechanics, why would one suppose that there may be no cognitive constraints in the case of *Homo sapiens*? What reason do we have to believe that for us, as opposed to our evolutionary ancestors, there are no fields of enquiry that are, in principle, closed or that there are no areas of cognitive closure?

Second, Carruthers claims that it does appear that McGinn has something importantly right: you cannot explain experience *directly* in terms of neurophysiological states of the brain. I agree. We saw that we cannot come up with the required conceptual connection by appealing to neurophysiological properties of the brain. But this, says Carruthers, may not be because experience is inherently inexplicable or because the explanation is cognitively closed to us, but rather because "we have pitched the explanation at the wrong level". Again, I agree. Carruthers writes:

> It may be that we have tried to jump over too many explanatory levels at once. Characterising the problem of phenomenal consciousness [what-it-is-likeness/experience] as a mind–brain problem, as is standardly done, is actually about as useful as characterising the problem of *life* as a life-sub-atomic-particle problem, or the problem of understanding the process of embryo development as the embryo-quark problem.   (2000: 90)

But there are indeed many different levels of scientific enquiry and description between neuroscience and folk psychology. To which level should we appeal for an explanation of experience? Carruthers thinks that the right general strategy to adopt is to attempt to explain experience in *cognitive terms*. Since experience is a mental phenomenon, we might as well appeal to cognitive or mental parts and processes to explain it, thus exploring the possibility of explaining experience in cognitive terms. Is such a higher-level explanatory strategy the key to the solution of the hard problem of consciousness? I think it is. In the remainder of this section, I shall sketch this strategy in light of our discussion so far, and in the following chapter I shall present in more detail the actualist HOT account that, I believe, can help us solve the explanatory gap problem.

We saw that both the idea of an outstanding epistemic gap and the appeal to ontological dualism are not satisfying enough: the first amounts roughly to "we do not know" or "we will never be in a position to know", and the second to introducing an extravagant doctrine and another explanatory gap. So what are we to do? I suggest a third option: although there are currently no known physical or neurophysiological facts in virtue of which we can reductively explain facts about experience, this is not to say that there are not any such facts that can do the explaining. There may be *non-experiential cognitive facts* that can fix an *a priori* conditional in the required sense. In other words, we may be able to establish a *conceptual connection* between non-conscious cognitive facts and experiential facts.[17]

It is indeed not clear whether cognitive or mental parts are to be allowed in a *reductive* explanation. This depends, of course, on how we are to understand the "levels" of explanation. However, in this case, we are explaining experiential facts by using non-experiential facts and, as Chalmers says, reductive explanation is explanation *wholly in terms of simpler* entities, that is, the explanatory premises of a reductive explanation of experience (or phenomenal consciousness in Chalmers's terminology) *must not refer or appeal to experience or facts that essentially require consciousness.* Cognitive parts that are themselves non-conscious (or that can be specified with no appeal to experience or facts that essentially require consciousness) make no appeal to experience or facts that essentially require consciousness. Therefore, the explanatory premises of a reductive explanation can include such cognitive facts.[18] This is further justified by the Chalmers (Chalmers & Jackson 2001) and Block (2002) view (see also Nagel 1974; Kim 2005) that experiential properties are distinct from any cognitive intentional or functional properties and that what makes the problem of consciousness hard, as opposed to the easy problems, is precisely that we cannot exhaustively explain it in terms of cognitive or intentional facts.

Of course, it is not a straightforward matter that non-conscious cognitive facts are themselves physical facts. In this sense, we do not show that P2 in the Chalmers and Jackson argument above (see p. 134) is false, since P2 requires that the left-hand side of the conditional be fixed by physical facts. At the same time, though, we do show that there is no reason to believe that we cannot reductively explain what-it-is-likeness or experience, since we can use non-experiential facts to establish the required conceptual connection. Here is the argument:

> If the left-hand side of the conditional in P1 does not include non-conscious cognitive facts, then P1 is false; if it does include such facts, then P2 is false because we can currently establish the required conceptual connection for experience by appealing to such facts.[19]

Strictly speaking, this will not close the explanatory gap since we have not yet shown that mental or cognitive facts are physical, but it will point towards a direction that looks very promising. Explanation of experience in terms of non-conscious cognitive properties does not require the postulation of any mysterious essentially conscious "phenomenal qualities" or "brute phenomenal facts", and it is not lying beyond human capacity (mystery). Recall that, according to Chalmers, the main reason that experience is the hard problem of consciousness is that "the easy problems are easy precisely because they concern the explanation of cognitive abilities and functions". Indeed, to explain a cognitive function, we need only specify a mechanism that can perform the function. As Chalmers puts it:

> the easy problems are the kind of problems that neuroscience and psychology can get at sort of straightforwardly … they're going to take a long time to solve, and they'll require a lot of intelligence, creativity and hard work. But we're gradually getting at these questions using the methods of neuroscience and psychology. It's slow work, but there is a clear sense that we have a research program there. We know roughly which direction to move in to get a result.   (See Jones 1996)

Chalmers has applied the term "easy" to problems that lie within the realm of physics, or at any rate science, for the very reason that these problems exhaustively concern the explanation of cognitive abilities and functions. Thus, if I am right, the hard problem of consciousness is not unlike the easy problems that lie in the realm of science. And clearly this is progress.

145

6 EXPERIENCE AND HIGHER-ORDER REPRESENTATIONALISM

6.1 HIGHER-ORDER REPRESENTATIONALISM

In the previous chapters we saw that there is good reason to think that mental qualitative properties are explanatorily irrelevant to experience or what-it-is-likeness. Further, we cannot come up with the required explanation for experience by appealing to any number of physical properties of neural states. Thus we should attempt a different explanatory strategy. Since consciousness is what makes mental states experiences – that is, such that there is something it is like for one to be in them – it could itself be a mental phenomenon, and since, as we saw previously, *dispositionalism* falls short of providing the required explanation, we need to appeal to *actualist* theories of consciousness.

Higher-order representationalist theories of consciousness hold that first-order representation does not suffice to account for the distinction between conscious and unconscious states. The answer to the question "What makes or transforms an unconscious mental state into a conscious one?" is, typically, some (higher-order) awareness of the state in question. According to higher-order representationalism (HOR), a state is a conscious state just in case *it is* or *is disposed to be* the object of a higher-order mental state. The latter is a state that represents or is about the lower (first-order) state, which is generally thought of as a perceptual or quasi-perceptual state.

There are several versions of HOR. The higher-order state – that is, the awareness required – can be a thought about the first-order state (HOT theory; e.g. Rosenthal 1991) or a kind of perception of the first-order state (Lockean or inner-sense theory; Lycan 1996). On both higher-order thought (HOT) and higher-order perception (HOP) accounts, that a mental state is conscious is a relational fact, requiring some additional mental state representing the first-order state in a suitable way. According to the HOT view, the higher-order state is a thought about the first-order state (e.g. sensory state), while on the HOP account a second-order sensory state is required: what it is like for one to be in a mental state is explained not in terms of a HOT but in terms of a second-order phenomenal or qualitative character.[1]

Generally, according to HOR, to say that there is something it is like for X (a subject) to be in Y (a mental state) is to say that X is conscious or aware of Y. To say that X is conscious of Y is to say that X is having a suitable HOT or HOP to the effect that X is in Y. Hence when one is in a conscious mental state – say one sees the cat on the mat – there is a higher-order mental state: one thinks or perceives oneself as seeing the cat on the mat. But only the first-order mental state need be a conscious state; there is something it is like to see the cat on the mat. The higher-order state need not be a conscious state; there need be nothing it is like to think or perceive oneself as seeing the cat on the mat.

A central commitment of most HOR theories (especially the HOT theories) is that they provide a *reductive explanation* of consciousness. Generally, reductive explanations are explanations wholly in terms of simpler entities, hence the name: reductive. A reductive explanation of consciousness will explain it wholly on the basis of principles or properties that do not themselves make any appeal to conscious properties. Hence if a HOR theory is to be reductive it must show – at least – that none of the abilities that one must possess for a suitable higher-order state to occur essentially requires consciousness. If these theories are to be reductive they must explain consciousness by reducing it to a relation between non-conscious states, namely mental states such that there is nothing it is like for one to be in them.

The main idea here is that, according to HOR, to say that a particular mental state of mine is conscious is to say that I am conscious or aware *of* it, but my awareness of a mental state does not itself have to be something I am conscious of. The first-order state is experienced by virtue of my awareness of it but this awareness need not be something I am aware of. But I can be aware of it (the second-order state) and that is roughly by virtue of a third-order state: further awareness to the effect that I am aware *of* being aware of a particular mental state.[2] Hence one can be in a conscious state (i.e. non-introspective) without being conscious of being in that state. To be conscious of being in that state would be to have introspective awareness of the consciousness of that state. There is a distinction to be drawn between three kinds of states: unconscious states, non-introspectively conscious states (first-order experiences) and introspectively conscious states (higher-order experiences). Using a small piece of notation here, we might say that if m is the first-order (unconscious) mental state then $A(m)$ is the non-introspectively conscious mental state (that is, one is aware that one is in m) and $A(A(m))$ is the introspectively conscious state (one is aware that one is aware of being in m).[3]

There are, however, other versions of HOR. Armstrong (1968), for instance, an advocate of the perceptual model, holds that one is conscious of a particular mental state only if one is introspectively aware of it by means of an inner sense. On this account, the above stated threefold distinction collapses into two, namely into non-conscious and introspectively conscious states.[4]

Armstrong is not alone in this. It appears that when we are non-introspectively conscious of a particular mental state, no unconscious higher-order state is revealed. (But this is not surprising since we are not aware of the higher-order state by virtue of which we are aware of this particular first-order mental state.) Hence, because our non-introspectively conscious states do not reveal any such higher-order states, many philosophers have concluded that no such thoughts occur at the non-introspective level. Carruthers (1996, 2000), for instance, holds that HO states, by virtue of which one is aware that one is in m, must be conscious; $A(m)$ must itself be a conscious state. Hence, on Carruthers's account, our threefold distinction sketched above collapses into a twofold distinction.

There is a problem with such accounts. These accounts face the obvious difficulty of generating a vicious infinite regress of nested conscious states. If the first-order state m being a conscious state is explained by a higher-order conscious state $A(m)$, then surely the higher-order state $A(m)$ being a conscious state itself requires explanation, presumably by a third-order conscious state $A(A(m))$. And now a regress is launched: one must be aware of being aware of being aware of being aware of being aware ... that one is in m (i.e. $A(m)$, $A(A(m))$, $A(... A(m) ...)$]. But on the above accounts (on the threefold distinction), $A(m)$ need not be itself a conscious state. So there is no danger of infinite regress on those accounts. The hierarchy does not extend beyond the first $A(m)$ for non-introspective experience, and extends for introspective experience only as far as our practical ability to think thoughts about our experiences, thoughts about thoughts about our experiences, and so on. And it is plain that when one is conscious of being in m one is not always conscious of being conscious that one is in m. There is no entailment from $A(m)$ to $A(A(m))$. Furthermore, on the threefold account, there is a clear distinction between consciousness and introspective consciousness.

Carruthers's way out of the predicament of the infinite regress of mental states is to suggest that only dispositions for HOTs to occur are necessary for non-introspectively conscious states. Carruthers thinks that this gets him out of the predicament since non-introspectively conscious states are conscious by virtue of being available to produce conscious HOTs, not by virtue of actually producing those thoughts. This does not produce a vicious infinite hierarchy of actual HOTs because a state need merely be disposed to cause a conscious HOT to be conscious itself. But it is not clear to how this can get him out of the predicament. Carruthers is still left with an infinite hierarchy of dispositions and, for one thing, it is hard to see how there can really be an infinite hierarchy of dispositions if only the first few ever get manifested.

This distinction – namely, that between a state being conscious in virtue of being *disposed* to give rise to a HOT (dispositional higher-order theory; Carruthers 2000) and being conscious by virtue of being the *actual target* of such a thought (actualist higher-order theory; Rosenthal 1991; Lycan 1996) – puts Carruthers's view in the category of first-order representationalism (FOR) since, according to him, some first-order states are sufficient for experience, that is, they merely have to be disposed to cause a HOT, not to cause such a thought. So on this account, no HOT need occur.[5]

There are two main models of actualist HOR accounts: HOP and HOT theory. We could become conscious of something by sensing or perceiving it or by virtue of having a suitable thought about it. I shall start by discussing the Lockean inner-sense or HOP view and I shall then look at the actualist HOT theory. We shall see that the latter can provide the required reductive explanation for experience. I shall address some of the standard objections to a HOT account of experience and conclude by exploring the relation between a HOT account and the idea that the content of our perceptual experiences is conceptual.

6.2 HIGHER-ORDER PERCEPTION THEORY

A traditional answer to the question of what it is that makes some of our mental states conscious is the Lockean idea that we become conscious of our mental states by some kind of "inner sense". According to the Lockean classical view, the perception of the operations of our own minds within us is not a *sense* since it has nothing to do with external objects; yet it is very like it, and might properly enough be called *internal sense*. What makes us aware of the mental states we are having is this sense: our introspective scanner. A motivation for this view is that the mental qualitative properties one is able to experience are not restricted by one's conceptual repertoire. As Gareth Evans (1982) put it, it appears implausible to suggest that we have a concept for every shade of colour we are able to discriminate. It appears that perceptual discrimination outstrips our conceptual repertoire. Thus, assuming that conceptual discrimination is more limited than perceptual discrimination, HOP theory appears to have an advantage over HOT theory in that it would seem that it can account for this assumption: no high-powered conceptual capacities are required for the production of HOPs. Thus it would seem that HOP theory can do something that HOT theory cannot: accommodate the rich detail of perceptual states.

However, HOP theory faces serious difficulties. An inner sense, for instance, would require an inner-sense organ or mechanism. Rosenthal writes:

> Since perceiving depends on a dedicated organ or mechanism, the [inner] perceptual model raises the question of what special organ or mechanism subserves being conscious of one's mental states. The absence of any such organ or mechanism may tempt one to conclude that being conscious must be something internal to conscious states [rather than something due to inner perception of the state].
> (1997: 750)

Rosenthal is not alone in holding this view (see also Dennett 1991a; Shoemaker 1994). A compelling reason to agree with Rosenthal is that it appears that the only mental qualitative properties that occur when mental states are conscious are those of the states of which we are conscious, and there are no additional qualities in virtue of which we are conscious of those states. Furthermore, there is no clear empirical evidence to suggest that there is such a neuro-mechanism. At the very least, then, the inner-sense theorist has an empirical obligation that is, as yet, unfulfilled.

But this is not the only objection to HOP theory. The perceptual model of awareness applies not only to non-introspective awareness but also to intro-spective awareness: there are two separate points depending on what kind of HOP variant one endorses. This has been another source of confusion in that some philosophers attack higher-order views to the effect that they cannot distinguish between consciousness and introspection or introspec-tive consciousness. On the actualist HOT theory account, the distinction is clear. Owing to the threefold distinction sketched previously, introspective consciousness is kept distinct from consciousness: a mental state is conscious by virtue of one's having a HOT to the effect that one is in that state, but intro-spection has nothing to do with it. The HOT need not itself be conscious. However, Armstrong, for instance, an advocate of the perceptual model, says that one is conscious of a particular mental state only if one is *introspectively aware* of it by means of an inner sense (1968). On this account the threefold distinction collapses into two: namely into non-conscious and introspectively conscious states. So in this case, it does matter whether there are reasons to believe in the *perceptual model of introspection*. On the other hand, one may hold that the inner sense operates only in the case of non-introspectively conscious states and that the perceptual model of introspection is false. There are two different versions of the HOP theory, and thus in what follows I shall address them both.

One of the most recent attempts to defend the perceptual model of intro-spection (PMI), a view that has fallen on hard times in the philosophy of mind, is by Gregg Elshof (2005). According to Elshof, the central theses that characterize an account of introspection that is a version of PMI are: (i) by introspecting, human beings are engaging in some form of reflection or *inner perception* of their own occurrent mental states; (ii) introspective access to these mental states is private; (iii) at least some first-level mental states exist independently of the subject's inner perception of them; and (iv) human beings sometimes acquire knowledge concerning their own mental states *by means of such inner perception* (*ibid.*: 23–4, emphasis added). As we would hope, Elshof takes care to draw a few distinctions such as the one between "inner" and "outer" perception. He says that the objects of introspection are "internal" in the sense that "there is *a way* of knowing about them which is available *only* to [the subject] S" (*ibid.*: 14). He admits that the postulated theses are compatible with competing models of introspection. What differentiates the perceptual model (inner-sense view) is this *way* of knowing, which is like sense perception. According to Elshof, we become introspectively aware by means of such inner perception.

However, Elshof rejects the view that it is an organ that does the observing when introspection occurs. What is it then? What is the nature of the inner perception or observation as opposed to outer perception? And why are we to hold on to the perceptual model of introspection? Elshof argues that looking at an object is not sufficient for attending. He claims that attention is a characteristic of inner (not just outer) perception, since one can attend, for instance, to one's memory of Neil Armstrong's first step on the moon or to one's memory of one's first day at school, which are not currently sense-perceptible. According to Elshof, the commonality between inner and outer perception is selective attention, and this is what grounds the perceptual model of introspection. But initially, you will recall, we wanted to know introspection's special *way* of knowing in the case of the inner-sense view. What we come to know is that this is not due to an inner-sense organ and that "self-knowledge is no *more* mysterious for being of something which is not sense perceptible since knowledge of sense perceptible features of the world requires the exercise of this same capacity" (*ibid.*: 91).

Elshof concludes with his less-than-satisfactory remark that it is not the case that sense organs do the attending in outer perception either, and therefore the same action of attending is required both for knowledge of empirical objects and for knowledge of our own cognitive operations. What is common between inner and outer perception is selective attention, and one does not need an inner organ for this because it is not the case that sense organs do the attending in outer perception either. Unfortunately, Elshof takes little care, if any, to explain "attention" and, in the case of outer perception, attention is arguably inextricably related with the operation of sense organs. Whereas it may be true that sense organs do not do the attending, whatever does it, could not do it without them. All in all, our thoughts possess the capacity for selective attention too, and, in the absence of any dedicated organ to be somehow related to this "inner perception" or any special kind of attention, it is hard to see why we should endorse PMI.

Lycan (1996, 2004), another propounder of the inner-sense view, has suggested that we have a set of inner-sense organs (attention mechanisms) charged with the scanning of the outputs of our first-order senses to produce HOPs of our own perceptual states. (Again, HOP theory does not explicitly depend on the existence of a dedicated organ to do the inner sensing.) Inner scanners produce higher-order perceptual representations in order to coordinate and relay information about mental states, and thus in order to better plan and monitor action. But besides the problem of how the mechanisms of evolution led to the construction of such inner scanners and the complexity of their operations, the HOP theorist needs to tackle another problem. One of the main objections to HOP theory is that even notebook computers, for instance, are self-scanning (Rey 1983). One less-than-satisfactory reply is that any such self-monitoring system may in fact possess a low degree of consciousness but there may be no determinate number of consciousnesses in a single body. A better reply is that there is an evolution-based constraint on consciousness, which is that only monitoring for the subject can contribute to consciousness (Lycan 1996). However, there is plausibly nothing it is like *for* a self-monitoring system such as a notebook to undergo a self-monitored state.

There are other problems for HOP. If the inner sense is substantially like our outer sense, should we not be able to doubt the testimony of the former in like manner? It seems implausible to suggest that one cannot doubt the testimony of the inner eye but can doubt the testimony of the outer. It may, for instance, appear to me that I see a green apple before me and I can doubt that there is a green apple before me. But this ought to hold for the inner eye as well. But it does not seem possible that I am able to doubt my seeming to see a green apple before me (think also of the Müller-Lyer illusion). What is more, as briefly mentioned, the presence of an inner sense implies the presence of some special higher-order qualities. Sensory modalities are distinguished by virtue of their distinctive qualitative properties. Sensations are classified by means of such properties and these in turn form sets or families of properties that pertain to colour, sound and so on. A higher-order perceptual mechanism would thus imply the existence of a distinctive family of qualitative properties uniquely associated with this mechanism. No such qualities appear to exist. There appears to be no qualitative characteristic aspect of the way we are conscious of our mental states. As Rosenthal puts the point, had such higher-order qualitative properties occurred in non-introspectively conscious states, were we to introspect those states we would be aware of them. And as introspection reveals, the qualities of the part of the sensory state that lights up by virtue of the higher-order state are the qualities by virtue of which we distinguish among different sensory modalities. What it is like for one to undergo a visual experience is not the same as what it is like for one to undergo an auditory experience. But it really depends on the distinctive qualitative properties that correspond with each of our (outer) sensory modalities. No qualities other than those that pertain to vision, audition and so on occur in our conscious qualitative states. The upshot is that perception (albeit higher-order) requires an associated manner of presentation, and there is none.

Additionally, it is hard to see how the inner-sense view can account for the cross-modal character of many of our perceptions. As Rosenthal has succinctly put the point:

> Since mental qualities are all specific to a single modality, higher-order sensing couldn't capture the cross-modal character that many of our perceptions exhibit. HOTs, by contrast, can readily operate across modalities. Since thoughts can have any content whatever, HOTs can make us conscious of perceptions in respect of all the mental qualities of a perception, whatever their modality. (2006: 203)

It appears, then, that HOP theory faces insurmountable difficulties. I should note that there remains the alleged problem for HOT theory that it cannot accommodate the idea that perceptual discrimination outstrips our conceptual repertoire. As we shall shortly see (§6.7), however, HOT theory is, in fact, far more plausible than HOP theory in this respect. Relatedly, HOP theory must somehow account for the fact that our perceptual experience becomes larger when we enlarge our conceptual capacities. We saw that the richer our conceptual repertoire, the more fine-grained the differences between the qualities of our sensory states. However, inner sense (or attention) may well have certain limitations. It does seem that, were we to have some sort of an inner organ, we could not enlarge our capacity for experience. All in all, it is hard to see how HOP theory can accommodate the idea that one enhances one's capacity for experience by enhancing one's conceptual repertoire.

6.3 HIGHER-ORDER THOUGHT THEORY

According to HOT actualist theories of consciousness (broadly construed), to say that there is something it is like for X (a subject) to be in Y (a mental state) is to say that X is conscious or aware of Y. Now to say that X is conscious of Y – and therefore experiences Y – is to say that X is having a suitable HOT to the effect that X is in Y. The idea, in the main, is that all manner of first-order mental states can occur unconsciously. Both first-order mental qualitative states (e.g. sensory states) and propositional attitudes (e.g. beliefs, desires, etc.) can occur unconsciously. This involves the idea that even mental states of the sort that possess the so-called qualia (being first order) can occur unconsciously. Hence, perceptual or sensory states (e.g. of the sort involved in seeing green and smelling the sea air), bodily sensations (e.g. feeling an itch) and felt emotions and moods (e.g. feeling delighted, depressed or tense) can occur unconsciously. Consciousness is a matter of there being something it is like for the subject to be in the state in question. The mental qualitative states that we are not aware of are not conscious: if one is not in any way aware of a mental state or that one is in that state then there is nothing it is like for one to be in it; if *one is not aware of* what it is like then there is nothing it is like *for one*.

One of the implications of this view is that the usual definition of qualia as being the properties in virtue of which there is something it is like for one to be in a mental state is mistaken. All manner of first-order states can occur unconsciously and hence there may be nothing it is like for one to be in them.[6] Hence we do not experience our mental states in virtue of the occurrence of mental qualitative properties. What makes certain mental states such that there is something it is like for one to be in them has nothing to do with whether or not a certain mental state is qualitative. We can, then, suggest that the same kind of awareness or consciousness can account for the experiential aspect of both conscious qualitative and conscious non-qualitative states (if there are any such states; e.g. propositional attitudes of the sort that do not involve any properties that are typically referred to as "qualia"). Following Rosenthal (1991, 2006), we can suggest that to say that a mental state is an experience or a conscious state is to say that one is conscious *of* or aware *of* that state and to say that one is conscious of that state is to say that one has a distinct (higher-order) state, that is, a HOT about this (first-order) state.[7] But the HOT in virtue of which one becomes conscious of a first-order state need not itself be conscious. This requires a third-order thought (introspection). This way, a theory of what it is to be conscious is kept distinct from a theory of what the objects of this consciousness are.

In my view, a HOT has the form "I am aware that p", where p is itself the report of a first-order mental state: either a mental qualitative state (e.g. "I am aware that either I am seeing or seeming to see a red patch") or a propositional attitude (e.g. "I am aware that I believe there is a red patch", or "I am aware that I believe that six sevens are forty-two"). Since all manner of first-order mental states can occur unconsciously, it would seem that there is no principled distinction between the two kinds of contents HOTs can have. But there does not have to be one, just a listing of cases. Thus we can say that mental qualitative states are states such as "I see a red patch or seem to see a red patch", "I hear a loud thud or seem to hear a loud thud", and so on for other sensory states, proprioceptive states, pains, itches, and so on. Propositional attitudes are states such as "I believe/doubt/wonder whether ... *p*". Now, in the case of a conscious qualitative state, the qualitative property must be part of the content of the HOT. I might, for example, be conscious of the solution to a mathematical problem, and the HOT might have only a mathematical content. Realizing this situation might be accompanied by pain or elation but these might be unconscious qualitative states, because there are no HOTs with those qualitative states as their contents. Of course, this requires the truth of the claim that mental qualitative states are not invariably or essentially conscious. In other words, if they are not part of the content of a HOT, there is nothing it is like for one to be in them.

Thus, HOTs are *intentional states* with a content and a mental attitude and not simply about an intentional content. To illustrate by means of an example, the truth conditions of statement (a) "it is raining" are not the same as the truth conditions of statement (b) "I think that it is raining". That is because (a) does not report a mental state; it is about the weather. And (b) reports a first-order thought. Now one who sincerely asserts (a) expresses a first-order thought (the thought that it is raining), and one who sincerely asserts (b) expresses a second-order thought (the thought that I think that it is raining). What requires consciousness is not the truth of what is asserted ((a) or (b)), since (a) may be true whether or not there is anything mental around, and (b) may be true but an unconscious belief. What entails consciousness is the truth of the HOT expressed (but not asserted) by "I think that it is raining". So when (b) is asserted, it is the truth of the HOT expressed (I think that I think that it is raining), not the first-order thought asserted (I think that it is raining) that implies that the speaker is conscious of the first-order thought: conscious of thinking that it is raining.

Further, HOTs are *unmediated*: they are not the product of inference. Mental states generate HOTs in an unmediated way and since mental states become conscious in virtue of an occurrent HOT, the HOT is unmediated.[8] We should also mention that mental states, as opposed to our physiological states, have the property of being potentially conscious, that is, they may not be essentially conscious, but are essentially *capable* of being conscious. The realization of this capacity is immediate: unmediated in that one can become conscious of a first-order mental state just by being in it, that is, mental states are *immediately sufficient* to generate HOTs. So, for instance, a mental qualitative state such as "I see or seem to see a red patch" and a propositional attitude such as "I believe that six sevens are forty-two" are mental states, but "I exercise too much" is not because the first two are each capable of immediately becoming the content of a HOT, whereas the latter is not (that I exercise too much is not *immediately sufficient* for "I am aware that I exercise to much").

Now, crucially, the higher-order representation represents the lower-order state as *a state of oneself*. In a Nagelian spirit, Rosenthal writes:

> Conscious[ness] of oneself ... must in any case occur if there is something it is like to have the experience. We're not interested in there being something it's like for somebody else to have the experience; there must be something its like *for one* to have it, oneself. Without specifying that, what it's like would be on a par with what it's like to be a table.   (2002a: 656, emphasis added)

Importantly, being conscious of ourselves in that way does not require that we are aware of ourselves in some privileged way that is antecedent to the HOTs we have about our own mental states: we said that a HOT makes one conscious of oneself as being in a particular mental state because it has the content that one is in that state. Hence, a HOT must somehow refer to oneself, but in what way? There is a famous case (Perry 1979) that runs as follows. Suppose that you are in a coffee shop and, looking through the window, notice somebody (more accurately, the reflection of a man) sitting alone, wearing a similar long black coat to yours and looking through the window, without realizing that this person is you. Your thought that "the man with the black coat is looking through this shop window" refers to you, but it does not refer to you as such. Suppose that you suddenly realize that the man in question is you. This time your thought is expressing a different proposition "I think I am looking through this shop window". In this case the indexical is essential. The HOT picks oneself out as the thinker of the first-order thought. A *de se* first-order thought that I am in *F* is not enough. Applied to John Perry's case, the switch is not *just* from "That man is looking through the window" to "I am looking through the window". By itself that is just a switch from one first-order thought to another. The idea is that the second *de se* thought disposes one to have a HOT: "I think I am looking through the window". What is required, then, is a HOT that identifies one as the thinker of that first-order thought: "I think I am in *F*" , that is, "It is me who thinks I am in *F*", and so on.

What does this essentially indexical self-reference consist in? The relevant thought picks out the individual who thinks this thought without *describing* the individual. The thought that "I am in *F*" disposes me to have another thought that *identifies* the individual the first thought is about as the thinker of that first thought. But this thought does not describe that individual, but only refers to it. The thought that *identifies* the individual the first thought is about *as the thinker of that thought* does not rest on an independent special access to the self. Essentially, indexical self-reference simply consists in the realization that the individual who looks through the window is the same as the individual who *thinks* that somebody looks through the window. Hence, essentially indexical self-reference requires no self-consciousness or any connection between first-order-person thoughts and the self.[9]

Essentially, indexical self-reference construed thus fits well with recent experimental findings. Gordon Gallup (1970) has shown that chimpanzees, for instance, but not monkeys, as well as children over eighteen months old, can recognize themselves in mirrors. Gallup used the following procedure. When a chimpanzee was anesthetized for its periodical medical check-up, an odourless red dye was applied to the chimpanzee's forehead while it lay unconscious. When the animal was awake again, a mirror was placed next to its cage, and the chimpanzee showed all the behaviours indicative of mirror self-recognition. The animal tried to wipe the dye from its forehead and it also positioned its body at various angles in front of the mirror in order to see places it could not ordinarily see on its own body.[10] This ability has been taken to imply the possession of a rudimentary "concept of self".[11] But this "concept of self" refers merely to the capacity of self-recognition or mirror recognition. Although we may (and there is no reason why we should not) suggest that these creatures have the ability for essentially indexical self-reference and they therefore can have HOTs and enjoy conscious qualitative states, this notion of recognition falls short of the most distinctive ability in human beings, which allows us to reflect on our mental lives and the mental lives of others. Self-consciousness requires this ability. Self-consciousness does not involve only the ability for self-reference or self-recognition. It involves an awareness of the ability for self-recognition and it is closely related with the concept of "personhood" that distinguishes us from other non-human animals. Self-consciousness requires the ability that enables us to attribute mental states in everyday life and to reflect on our mental lives and the mental lives of others.[12]

Summing up, then, non-introspectively conscious states require HOTs that need not be themselves conscious. The core requirement of such HOTs is that they must represent the first-order states as states of oneself. The "'of oneself" requirement amounts to the ability for self-reference, which in turn does not require self-consciousness or any introspective capacities. We also saw that the HOTs in virtue of which we are non-introspectively conscious are not themselves conscious. This is because we are not conscious of them, and for a mental state to be conscious is for one to be conscious of it. Granted that all manner of first-order mental states can occur without there being anything it is like for the subject to be in them, we have specified all the requirements of such a non-conscious HOT with no reference or appeal to experience or facts that essentially require consciousness. None of the abilities that one must possess for a suitable HOT to occur essentially require consciousness. And, arguably, genuine explanations work by drawing connections between a set of facts (what does the explaining) and a distinct set of facts (what needs explaining). Our explanation then satisfies that criterion since the connection is drawn between non-conscious cognitive facts and experiential or conscious facts.

6.4 CLARIFYING THE PROPOSAL

We started from Nagel's idea that to be a conscious creature is to be such that there is something it is like *for that creature* to be that creature. For example, for John to be consciously seeing a red patch, there is something it is like *for John* to be seeing a red patch, where that "for John" involves Perry's self-ascribing indexical. This is best captured by ascribing to John a higher-order belief expressed from John's point of view as: I believe I am seeing a red patch. The hard problem of consciousness is, according to Chalmers, to explain the phenomenon of conscious experience in purely naturalistic terms. Responses to this challenge vary widely. Chalmers himself thinks no such explanation is possible unless we add proto-consciousness to our basic inventory of natural categories. McGinn holds that the explanation exists in Platonic heaven, so to speak, but is beyond our ken. I think that taking experience to essentially involve such higher-order thought, when suitably developed, renders the explanatory reduction of consciousness in naturalistic terms tractable.

It is commonplace that first-order propositional attitudes need not be conscious. More recently it has been recognized that first-order perceptual states too need not be conscious: a blindsight patient may see a cross on the paper, as evidenced by their regularly correct "guesses", as they would say, when there is nothing it is like for them, in Perry's proprietary sense of "for them", to see the cross. Now, the possibility of unconscious perception is recognized. We saw that it is commonplace and widespread. A competent motorist driving in undemanding conditions may ease her foot from the accelerator slightly as she sees the car ahead slow for the bend, but need not be conscious of seeing such, her attention being on the urgent conversation with her passenger on quite other matters. First-order propositional attitudes and perceptual states *per se*, I have argued, do not require consciousness.

When we add HOTs the picture changes, but *not* immediately. Our blindsight patient sees the cross on the paper, but not consciously so. He may come, when he finds himself disposed to "guess" there is a cross, to believe that he sees the cross because the experimenter, whom he trusts, tells him so. Or becoming knowledgeable about his condition he forms a theory that when he is inclined to "guess" cross it is because he is seeing a cross. But the advent of such higher-order beliefs does not cure his blindsight; he still does not consciously see the cross. Nor would it be enough for the higher-order belief to come to him spontaneously and without rational ground. For it is conceivable that some future investigator might be able to induce that higher-order belief in our patient spontaneously and without it having a rational ground from the patient's viewpoint, just by pressing a button that activates directly appropriate nodes in his belief area, so our patient, as well as having the inclination to plump for the answer "cross", also finds himself believing that he sees it, as he did formerly on the experimenter's testimony, while yet not consciously seeing it. I suggest that what we need to constitute consciously seeing the cross, what we need for there to be something that it is like for him, in Perry's proprietary sense, to be seeing the cross, is for him to believe that he is seeing the cross *on the rational ground of his being visually aware of the cross*. I mean the italicized phrase in such a way that it *conceptually implies* (entails) visual consciousness of the cross. (I do not take it to conceptually imply [entail] consciousness of the higher-order propositional attitude itself.)

This is the explanandum for which we seek naturalistic reductive explanans. It is not the explanans of consciousness, but the canonical description of what it is to be conscious, of what it is for there to be something it is like for one to be in that state, for which we seek a naturalistic explanation, where that naturalistic explanation may include first-order attitudes and perceptions that can themselves be explained in terms of naturalistic cognitive architectures. The task is beyond us at present, but it does not seem intractable. The task is to identify in nature, or to devise, a naturalistic cognitive architecture such that the subject sees a red patch, say, and believes that he sees a red patch, and the first cognitive state is from the subject's point of view the immediate rational ground of the second: the subject does not, from his point of view, have the belief groundlessly, nor have it on such indirect grounds as the testimony of the experimenter or the subject's own internalized theory of blindsight, whereby his inclination to guess becomes for him a symptom of his seeing. That is all on the side of the explanandum.

On the side of the explanans, this seems a matter of the *kind* of causal connection between the first-order belief and the higher-order belief that it causes. We want a characterization of a path that is normal and epistemically appropriate in the circumstances the creature inhabits for the formation of higher-order beliefs that serve in its cognitive ecology whatever function such beliefs normally serve, and that are from the subject's point of view immediately grounded by their content, not groundless and not the output of the subject's theorizing. Of course we cannot do this yet, and of course there are notorious difficulties here of identifying normal from deviant causal chains. But they do not seem to me problems of an insurmountable kind. I do not see the problem of giving a reductive explanation of consciousness as lying beyond human capacity (mystery) nor as requiring the addition of some proto-conscious element to our basic naturalistic categories.

My solution to the "hard" problem of consciousness is to reduce it to an "easy" problem. Taking an example of a conscious perceptual state – say, John consciously seeing a red patch – we can analyse it in terms of some condition C that does not mention consciousness and which satisfies the following two conditions:

(1) C is metaphysically sufficient (and necessary) for John consciously seeing a red patch. This comes down to claiming that it is inconceivable that John satisfy C with respect to a red patch, but not be consciously seeing a red patch. And vice versa, rather more tentatively, it is inconceivable to be consciously seeing a red patch, but C not hold.
(2) The elements in C are themselves amenable to functional explanation, thereby presenting only the "easy" problem.

The proposal I suggest for C is the following:

> John *consciously* sees a red patch (i.e. there is something it is like for John to see a red patch) if and only if:
> (a) John sees a red patch; and
> (b) John believes that he sees or seems to see a red patch;[13] and
> (c) (a) is his *direct warrant* (ground) for (b).

Plausibly this meets condition (1): (a) alone is clearly not sufficient (blindsight, the competent driver, cases of unconscious perception). Our blindsighted subject, for example, may satisfy analogues of (a) and also of (b) on the testimony of a trusted experimenter, but does not thereby consciously see that there is a cross in his right field, say. He may even come, as an experienced and knowing experimental subject, to trust his hunches: to believe, without prompting from the experimenter, when he feels inclined to report that he sees a cross, that he does indeed see a cross, thus spontaneously satisfying analogues of (a) and (b). But again, his blindsight is not thereby cured. His belief has the wrong kind of warrant: an indirect warrant rather than a direct perceptual warrant. In contrast, if he says "I believe I am seeing a red patch" on the most direct grounds possible, namely because he sees a red patch, then I cannot conceive of it not being the case that he *consciously* sees the red patch. So (a), (b) and (c) are metaphysically *sufficient* for John seeing a red patch.

But are (a), (b) and (c) metaphysically *necessary* for John consciously see-ing a red patch? At first sight it may appear not. I agreed that John may consciously see a red patch without his being aware of (b) nor therefore of (c). But, given the dispositional nature of belief, that is consistent with (b) and (c) being nonetheless true, without John being aware that he has this belief and that his belief has that warrant. If John consciously sees a red patch, then arguably John may become aware that he satisfies (b) when he is prompted, for example by the question: "Do you believe that you are seeing a red patch?" And having been so prompted, he may become aware that he satisfies (c) when he is prompted, for example by the further question: "Why do you believe that you are seeing a red patch?" Then he will be aware that he has the belief and that it is not ungrounded, but is directly grounded by experience of its content. This suggests that a case could be made that (a), (b) and (c) are together metaphysically *necessary* for John consciously seeing a red patch, even if John is not conscious of satisfying (b) or (c).

Regarding condition (2), we can take (a) and (b) to be straightforwardly amenable to (long arm) functional explanation. And, arguably, (c) is amena-ble to functional explanation. If we design a machine to have beliefs about its own states, then we will want those beliefs in the normal working of the machine to be rationally grounded, and the most direct canonical ground will be the presence of the state itself. A few more words about (c): I define a *direct warrant* for a belief that *p* as the fact that *p*. Thus if someone says "I believe I see (seem to see) a red patch" and we ask, "Why do you believe that?" in the relevant cases, the only correct answer is "Because I see (seem to see) that there is a red patch". This is a direct warrant. Similarly for nega-tive direct warrants: if someone says "I believe I see (seem to see) that there is no red patch" and we ask, "Why do you believe that?" in the relevant cases, the only correct answer is "Because I see (seem to see) that there is no red patch". Compare "I believe that God exists". We ask, "Why do you believe that?", and the answer is given, "Because God exists". The believer is claiming a direct warrant. The claim of a direct warrant is not trivial, since in percep-tual cases the believers do have such warrants, and their beliefs are rational, but the theist does not: claiming a direct warrant does not make the theist belief rational.[14]

A warrant for a belief should not be confused with the degree of confi-dence one may have in that belief. A warrant bestows *epistemic standing* on a belief, whereas a degree of confidence is a psychological state. The rela-tion between warrant and degree of confidence is complex. One may have a very high degree of confidence in one's belief that this lottery ticket will not win (the ticket being one of over twenty million sold), far higher than in one belief's that today is Tuesday, and this is even rational confidence: the chance of a given ticket winning is far, far lower than the frequency with which one mistakes the day of the week. But the belief that it did not win is not war-ranted until after the draw is known, whereas normally one's belief that it is Tuesday is warranted.

If a higher-order belief is so warranted then the belief is knowledge: *S* *knows* that she sees (seems to see) a red patch. A necessary condition for such a higher-order belief to be knowledge is that the warrant be reliable in the sense explored by reliabilist accounts of knowledge. (I do not claim that being reliable is also sufficient for knowledge, nor that reliability is a neces-sary condition for all kinds of knowledge – e.g. mathematical knowledge. So I am not committing myself to a reliabilist account of warrants in general, nor to an analysis of warrants.)

Finally, notice that on this account there are no similar mental-causation problems. There is no reason to worry about a spatial–non-spatial causal relation. As in the case of water, where the behaviour of H_2O molecules at 212°F at sea level does not *cause* boiling (or the properties of the H_2O mol-ecules do not *cause* liquidity in normal conditions), this pattern of cognitive activity does not *cause* experience. The boiling of water simply *consists in* a certain activity of H_2O molecules at 212°F at sea level. In like manner, being conscious of a mental state (which makes that state an experience) consists in having a suitable HOT – higher-order warranted belief – about it. We do not need to postulate boiling as a process separate from the loosening of the H-bonds. If we identify them we get a smooth explanation. Similarly, if we separate first- and second-order mental states, and identify what-it-is-likeness with HOTs, we get a smooth explanation of those cases where we do want to attribute consciousness and those where we do not. My proposal, then, is along the same lines as the *reductive explanation* of boiling in terms of H-bond loosening (see Chalmers & Jackson 2001): not a logical deduction, but an argument to the best explanation.[15]

6.5 NON-CONSCIOUS AND NON-VITAL ZOMBIES

It should be of interest to contrast the mystery of experience with the mystery of life. It is a well-known fact that although the scientific understanding of the biochemical processes that distinguish living from non-living matter has become increasingly sophisticated, so has the realization that these funda-mental processes are incredibly complicated. It is striking that no complete, reductionist theory has yet been proposed that coordinates all the actions that occur in a single cell (let alone a higher organism). No known law of physics or scientific principle suggests an inbuilt drive from matter to life or the emergence of the living state over other states. Even in terms of the biol-ogy of the cell itself, life cannot currently be accurately described simply by understanding any number of chemical processes that occur in the cell. To put the point differently, life cannot currently be *deduced* by any number of chemical processes in the cell. We are not in position to solve the problem of life by appealing to physics and chemistry.

Are we, then, to postulate *élan vital* – some special mysterious stuff or vital spirit – as a fundamental property of nature alongside mass, force and, presumably, proto-experience to solve the problem? No. This is not how we now think about life. Chemical and anatomical discoveries pushed aside the "vital force" or *élan vital* explanation, as more and more life processes came to be described in purely scientific terms, and as the medical model of disease came to be increasingly focused on the failure of particular organs and processes in the body. In so far as all biological functions and processes – such as reproduction, development, growth, metabolism, self-repair and immunological self-defence – are filled in there is nothing left over to be explained. In the case of life too, therefore, we have come to accept a reductive explanation. There is nothing left over to be explained because, in the case of a particular organism, its being alive consists in such and such physico–chemical homeostatic processes.

Similarly, as it is widely accepted, experience cannot currently be deduced by any number of neurophysiological processes in the brain or properties of neurons. But as in the case of life, this does not mean that experience cannot be entailed by any number of (cognitive) functions and biological processes. It just means that we hit the wrong level of explanation and that we should dismiss some of our mistaken assumptions about experience. Leaving aside the idea that our mental qualitative properties or qualia somehow carry consciousness within themselves, I see no more reason to postulate anything like proto-experience as a fundamental property of nature to solve the problem of experience. We just need to appeal to a different level of explanation: in the case of life we had to appeal to the biological level. In the case of experience, we must appeal to the cognitive level.

It might be objected that we can still coherently imagine that there is a living organism that is functionally and behaviourally indistinguishable from a conscious one (with which they share the same environment and have the same causal histories), with which you can have a meaningful conversation and which has a HOT of the kind described above, for example, a warranted belief to the effect that it realizes (veridically self-ascribes) that a solution to a problem goes a certain way without thereby being anything it is like for the organism to be in that state (is not conscious). But contrast the case of a non-conscious with a non-vital zombie. Can we, for instance, imagine something that is capable of reproduction, development, growth, metabolism, self-repair and immunological self-defence, but that is not alive? If the answer is yes, then, as Dennett puts the point, this shows only "that you can ignore 'all that' and cling to a conviction if you're determined to do so" (1991a: 281–2).[16]

6.6 THE PROBLEM OF THE ROCK

A few years ago, Alvin Goldman wrote:

> How could possession of a meta-state confer subjectivity of feeling on a lower-order state that did not otherwise possess it? Why would being an intentional object or referent of a meta-state confer consciousness on a first-order state? A rock does not become conscious when someone has a belief about it. Why should a first-order psychological state become simply by having a belief about it? (1993: 266)

This is called the "problem of the rock". The standard reply by HOR theorists, in a nutshell, is this: first-order mental states are psychological states and rocks are not. There are certain features that make certain states of the organism mental. These features are not to be found even in *internal* physiological states such as liver states. Hence, there is something special not only about the meta-conferring consciousness state, but also about the first-order state. And as Rocco Gennaro puts the point, "after all, the HOT theory is attempting to explain *what makes a mental state* a conscious mental state" (2005: 6).[17]

But we have not yet solved the problem of the rock. For Goldman here wants to know exactly *how* or *why* these meta-states can confer consciousness on their objects. That is, exactly *how* does having a HOT directed at a mental state make that state conscious or such that there is something it is like for one to be in it? This bears a striking resemblance to Chalmers's "hard" problem of consciousness: even if we agree that that HOTs confer consciousness to first-order mental states, we have no good explanation of why and how they do it. And I think Gennaro here gives an unsatisfactory answer. Here is what he says

> The solution, then, is that HOTs explain how consciousness arises because the *concepts* that figure into the HOTs are presupposed in conscious experience … In very much a Kantian spirit, the idea is that first we passively receive information via the senses. Some of this information will then rise to the level of unconscious mental states … But such mental states do not become conscious until the "faculty of understanding" operates on them via the application of concepts. (*Ibid.*: 10)

He adds that "the concepts that we have clearly color the very experiences we have and removing all of them would eliminate the experience itself. Indeed, having such concepts on the HOT theory is both necessary and sufficient for having subjective conscious experience" (*ibid.*: 11). I agree that HOTs are conceptually structured and I do think that the content of conscious mental states is conceptual. But I fail to see how exactly this can be both a necessary and a sufficient condition for "subjective conscious experience".[18] As Gennaro himself later in the paper admits, "this is an adequate answer to the above challenge" (*ibid.*). One can ask: why does this higher-order application of concepts give rise to conscious experience? Gennaro replies:

> But, this I suggest, is not a legitimate question. We have already reached the rock bottom brute fact about the way that conscious minds work, and the chain of explanation has already come to an end. The Kantian idea that concepts make our experience of the world possible is surely a widely held view about the nature of conscious experience. I do not think that it makes sense to ask why this is so. (*Ibid.*: 11)

Well, it does. If I understand it correctly, the point at issue here is not to ask "*What* makes (conscious) experience possible?" but "*How* does it make – whatever *it* is – (conscious) experience possible?" For an answer to the first question could simply be "a HOT", and this way we are back to square one. As Gennaro himself admits at the start of his paper, the HOT theory is attempting to explain *what* makes a mental state a conscious mental state.

Here is what we might say. Nagel articulated his notion of "what-it-is-likeness" as follows:

> [W]hatever may be the status of facts about what it is like to be a human being, or a bat, or a Martian, these appear to be facts that *embody a particular point of view*. The facts about consciousness are *perspectival* in the sense that our conscious experiences have an inbuilt perspectival character; they embody a particular point of view. (1974: 441, emphasis added)

The facts about what-it-is-likeness then are perspectival in the sense that our experiences "embody a particular point of view". We want to know what it is like *for me* to be in a certain mental state, not for you or anyone else. An explanatory account of experience, then, must explain this "perspectivity" or "point of view". I suggest that self-ascription of the kind described above is essentially what characterizes non-introspectively conscious states (first-order experiences) and explains their perspectival character. As Kant puts the point in the *Critique of Pure Reason*, "it must be possible for the 'I think' to accompany all my representations, for otherwise … the representation … would be nothing to *me*" (1929: B 131, emphasis added). Following Kantian considerations, I suggested that self-ascription (self-reference or self-identification) and self-consciousness are distinct. Self-ascription does not require (or presuppose) self-consciousness. This way we avoid circularity. At the same time, self-ascription is what bestows our experiences with their perspectival character. When one recognizes oneself, one has a conception of oneself as embedded in an objective world; the subject represents himself as being embedded in an objective world. Employing the Nagelian jargon, we can say that the ability for self-recognition enables one to embody a particular "point of view". Self-ascriptions are then what enables the subject to embody a particular point of view of the world and makes the subject's mental states experiences, that is, mental states *for the subject*. The ability for self-ascription or self-recognition is a cognitive ability that many non-human primates have. And explanations of cognitive abilities and functions lie in the domain of science.[19]

In this connection, it is worth quoting Chalmers on this very idea of self-ascription:

> Zombie Dave ascribes precisely the same mental states to himself as I do! … How can this ability for self-ascription be explained? Clearly not by appealing to qualia, for Zombie Dave does not have any. The story will presumably have to be told in purely functional terms. But once we have this story in hand, it will apply equally to proud possessors of qualia such as ourselves. The self-ascription mechanisms that Zombie Dave uses are equally the mechanisms that we use; at most, *the difference consists in the fact that his ascriptions might be wrong, whereas ours are right* …
>
> (1993: 36, emphasis added)

Chalmers admits that there may indeed be a difference between self-ascription and zombie self-ascription: only the first is veridical. But unmediated HOTs cannot misrepresent. The higher-order warranted belief of the form "I believe that I see or seem to see a red patch" cannot be false. In cases of alleged misrepresentation, HOTs do not represent us as being in states that we are not actually in (*contra* Rosenthal). If an unmediated HOT, of the kind required, represents us as being in a certain first-order state, then we are in that state, we are having that experience. Since such a HOT does not misrepresent its first-order state, having the higher-order belief guarantees that I am not a zombie.[20]

6.7 EXPERIENCE, HOTS AND CONCEPTUALIZATION

In this section, I shall consider the question of whether perceptual experience has a non-conceptual content. This question has been vigorously debated for more than twenty years. The question has generated this much discussion because the possibility of non-conceptual content is intimately related not only with certain important aspects of the "hard problem", but also with fundamental issues in philosophy such as the relations between experience, belief and knowledge, the relations between experience and introspection, and the phenomenology of experience and its relations to the intentionality of experience.

I shall start this section by explaining the relevant terminology and I will then address some of the standard objections to the idea that perceptual experience has a conceptual content, including the objection from the *fineness of grain* of perceptual experience. Peter Carruthers (2000), for instance, urges that an occurrent thought would make us conscious of all the fine-grained distinctions among our visual experiences only if we had a concept for each just-discriminable shade of colour. The complaint is that, assuming that conceptual discrimination is more limited than perceptual discrimination, a HOT theory seems not to be able to account for the richness of our perceptual experiences. However, as we shall shortly see, an actualist HOT theory not only has the resources to meet this objection, but it also provides useful insights that can lead to a better understanding of the relevant phenomena.

According to most philosophers, perceptual experiences are conscious qualitative states that have accuracy conditions: they are accurate in certain circumstances and inaccurate in others. Perceptual experiences are by their nature such that *they present the world as being a certain way* and therefore are assessable for accuracy. But if one thinks that perceptual experiences have representational content, then one thinks of them as belief-like in some respects: Believing, for instance, that there is a piece of paper on the table, is being in a state with representational content. So how far can we push the analogy between perceptual experiences and beliefs? Do they, for instance, have the same *kind* of representational content?

The central idea behind the theory of non-conceptual content is that some mental states can represent the world and the subject of those mental states need not possess the concepts required to specify their content. It is notoriously difficult to give a positive characterization of non-conceptual content. The general idea is that, granted that the content of thoughts and beliefs is conceptual, we want to see whether the contents of perceptual experiences are as well. According to conceptualism, for instance, if two perceivers were looking at the same scene in the same conditions, but they each possessed different concepts for the features present in the scene – they have different conceptual repertoires – they would have visual experiences with different (representational) contents. Non-conceptualists deny this. *Contra* conceptualism, one's experience of the world is not constrained by one's conceptual capacities.

What is a "concept"? Recall Frege's example that the ancients did not know that the descriptions "The Morning Star" (or Phosphorus) and "The Evening Star" (Hesperus) referred to the same heavenly body, namely Venus. When they discovered it they learned something important: "The Morning Star is the Evening Star". This last statement is informative. It is informative because "The Morning Star" and "The Evening Star" have different intensions or meanings (senses). But they have the same extension (reference) – the thing or the set of things to which the term refers – that is, both refer to the same object, to the same heavenly body. I shall take it that a concept can be viewed as a Fregean sense (or mode of presentation) singling out a relation or an object-property in the world (e.g. roundness or the property of being a horse). The parallel to be drawn is with the linguistic expressions as they do also have sense and reference. Each concept has an extension, that is, it expresses a condition of reference and it refers to whatever satisfies that condition.

Within a Fregean tradition, the contents of propositional attitudes (e.g. beliefs) are taken to consist of concepts and it is hard to see how one can stand in a relation to a complex of concepts without possessing each of them. Gareth Evans's (1982) *generality constraint* provides us with a key to what we mean by the claim that beliefs have conceptual content. According to the generality constraint:

> no thinker is capable of entertaining a Thought with a particular structure unless she is able to recombine the elements of that structure so as to form other, related Thoughts. Note the mention here of a Thought's structure: I take it that it is this idea, that Thoughts are, in a certain sense, structured … if we call the elements of the structure "concepts", then we can put this point by saying that Thoughts are composed of concepts or, better, that Thoughts are conceptually articulated.   (Heck 2000: 487)

So to entertain the thought that Tom is tall (*Fa*), one must exercise the capacity to think of Tom and a capacity to think of a thing as being tall. Similarly, to entertain the thought that Mary is bright (*Gb*) one must exercise similar capacities. Now according to the generality constraint, if a subject can think that *Fa* and that *Gb*, then the subject must also have the capacity to think that *Ga* and that *Fb* (recombine the elements). So, then, to say that some mental states have non-conceptual content is to say that they are not conceptually articulated in the relevant sense. If perceptual experiences, for instance, have non-conceptual content, this means that "being in a perceptual state with a given content need not require one to grasp certain concepts (as determined by its content, namely, those of which its content is composed)" (*ibid*.: 488).

An important issue (in effect) is raised as to what individuates a given concept. Christopher Peacocke has postulated a criterion that, when met (satisfied), individuates a concept. He calls it a *possession condition*. A concept is individuated by its possession condition: the concept is the given one and not any other concept when it is individuated by "The condition which must be satisfied if a thinker is to possess that concept and to be capable of having beliefs and other attitudes whose contents contain it as a constituent" (1993: 74).

We might say, then, that one possesses a concept when one manages to individuate that concept by satisfying the possession condition. Thus, we may say that X is a concept if and only if it is a Fregean sense and a thinker that possess X satisfies its possession condition, so that X is a constituent of the intentional contents of judgements and beliefs of the thinker.[21]

You will recall that a belief is a representational state that consists of an attitude and a content (the intentional or representational "object") and hence there are two things that distinguish one representational state from another: the attitude and the content. As Mike Martin (1992) points out, if one claims that perceptual experiences have representational content that does not commit one to identifying experience with beliefs. Perceptual experiences will have the same kind of content as beliefs if: (a) experience is the same kind of attitude as belief; or (b), if (a) is false, then they are both attitudes to the same *kind* of content. In the discussion that follows, I shall be mostly focusing on (b). First, however, I shall briefly touch on (a).

It has been argued that owing to cases of "known" illusions, (a) cannot be true. Take the case of the Müller-Lyer illusion (Figure 6.1). We all know that the two horizontal lines are of equal length. But knowing this does not change the experience: one of the lines looks longer than the other, no matter what we believe about their length. Hence it might be suggested that that a visual experience of a Müller-Lyer diagram is independent of background belief, that is, its content does not *vary* or change with relevant background belief. As Kathrin Pagin (2009) points out, on the assumption that experi-

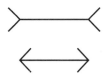

Figure 6.1 Geometric illusion designed by F. C. Müller-Lyer. The horizontal lines are the same length in both images. However, the horizontal line in the upper image seems to be longer.

ences are beliefs, independence from background belief thus leads to the conclusion that subjects of known illusions have contradictory beliefs. The problem seems to be that when one becomes aware of the illusion and the illusion persists, then, at a certain time t, if experiences were beliefs one would find oneself having contradictory experiences, that is, one would believe that p and *not-p* at the same time. However, as Pagin argues in the same paper, it is open to hold that the beliefs are not contradictory because the subject at t holds that "*X is F*", that is, "the *lines* are of equal size" and that "*X looks* not-*F*", that is, "the lines *look* unequal"; one can think at a certain time, for instance, that "the snow *is* white, but it *looks* not-white" (owing to unusual conditions of illumination). Hence, the contradiction disappears. This solution involves assuming that the content of the experience is that something *looks* a certain way (not that it is that way).

Now, what about (b)? We think of beliefs as conceptual states. The possession of a belief rests in one's capacities to think about objects and properties. As Martin (1992) asks, could our experiences be conceptual in this way: the appearance of things being restricted by one's conceptual capacities? Well, there is a striking connection between what thoughts we are able to have and what mental qualitative properties we are able to be aware of. In other words, it appears that *the content of our perceptual experiences varies with conceptual sophistication*. Our perceptual experience, for instance, becomes larger when we enlarge our conceptual capacities. Learning about music theory enables us to hear chords differently and with more richness and learning a bit more about gymnastics enables us to see the gymnast's exercises differently and with more detail. The same considerations hold regarding wine tasting or appreciating a work of art: the more rich our conceptual repertoire, the more fine-grained the differences between the qualities of our sensory states.

It is further suggestive that recent empirical findings (Rolls 2005) show that higher-order brain processing can influence perception of smell at its most primitive level. Rolls presented an ambiguous odour, which, according to him, might have been thought to be Brie but was labelled either "cheddar cheese" or "body odour". What happened was that the subjects rated the smell as much more pleasant when it was labelled cheese. And in magnetic resonance images, brain regions involved in early olfactory processing were activated more strongly by the positive label. Rolls concluded that language can reach down into our emotional system.

This case suggests that what-it-is-like for one to be in a particular mental qualitative state is determined by the way one is conscious of being in that state. Such cases exhibit an intimate relation between experience and one's conceptual capacities. They suggest that our beliefs can directly influence and determine our experiences; what it is like for one to be in a certain mental qualitative state is determined by the way that one's HOT represents that state. Both the learning capacity and Rolls's experiments suggest that our conceptual sophistication determines the content of our perceptual experiences and that our HOTs are of overriding significance. As Rosenthal puts it:

> So which contents our intentional states can have must somehow make a difference to which sensory qualities can occur consciously. Moreover, the new concepts, which make possible conscious experiences with qualities that seem new to us, are the concepts of those very qualities. [We can focus introspectively on the distinguishing properties of our conscious sensory states.] So being able to form intentional states about certain sensory qualities must somehow result in our being able to experience those qualities consciously. (2002b: 413)

On the account I am proposing, there is a distinction to be drawn between *perceptual experiences* and (unconscious) *perceptual states* in the sense that there is nothing it is like for one to be in the latter (which are nevertheless qualitative). In my view, all qualitative aspects of a *conscious* qualitative state are such that we have concepts of them. In other words, they are captured conceptually. But notice that this view leaves room for us to hold that the content of our perceptual states (non-experiential) is non-conceptual. It is one thing to claim that the content of perceptual experience is conceptual and it is another to claim that the content of our (unconscious) perceptual states is (I remain neutral about the latter). However, I do think that the content of our perceptual experiences is conceptual (the content of HOTs). A HOT conceptualizes the first-order content, because it is a propositional attitude to the first-order state: I believe that I see a red patch. What follows the "believe", "that I see a red patch", refers to a proposition, a conceptual entity. Hence, on my view, the qualities of which someone can be conscious are limited by their conceptual repertoire. I should add that it is not the higher-order element of the HOT that contains the conceptualization of the first-order qualitative state, since the higher-order element is common to all the relevant HOTs, namely, I believe that *p*. It is the first-order element of the HOT that conceptualizes the first-order qualitative state: "I believe that I see a red patch", in contrast to, say, "I believe that I hear a blackbird sing".

Most philosophers talk about the content of perceptual experience and the content of perceptual states interchangeably (e.g. Martin 1992; Peacocke 2001).[22] This is a mistake. Even if it turns out that perceptual content (unconscious) is non-conceptual, it does not follow that the content of perceptual experience (conscious) is also non-conceptual. We saw earlier that recent empirical findings strongly suggest that there are unconscious sensory states;

namely, mental qualitative states of which we are not in any way aware. This fits well with our distinction and with the widely held view that perceptual content (non-experiential) is non-conceptual. As it turns out, one can hold both that the content of our perceptual experiences is conceptual and that the informational richness of the content of our perceptual states cannot be matched by the conceptual content of our thoughts. Interestingly, the non-conceptual content of our perceptual states is linked with the requirements of our bodily actions (Peacocke 1992) or with the linkages between sensory and motor systems that explain how action can be perceptually guided. Non-conceptual content is linked with what some philosophers (O'Regan & Noë 2001) call "sensorimotor contingencies"; namely, regularities in the way that sensory stimulation changes as a result of movement by the agent and by objects in the environment. Recall that it is the *non-conscious* dorsal-stream processing that is associated with our perceptual sensorimotor system.[23] According to the account I am proposing, then, since the subject is unaware of such processing the content of those states is not experienced (i.e. it is not conscious). Hence, it is open to hold that the content of those mental states is non-conceptual. Therefore, the idea that the content of perceptual experience is conceptual remains intact from the claim that the informational richness of our perceptual content transcends our conceptual capacities.

Furthermore, according to some non-conceptualists, what it means to say that a mental state M of a subject Y has non-conceptual content C at t_1 is that C is not part of the content of Y's beliefs and thoughts at t_1. This fits well with the experimental findings I cited in Chapter 3. Recall, for instance, the phenomenon of change blindness, where very large changes occur in full view in a visual scene (in visual perception) but are not noticed. Recall also Repp's perceptual-motor synchronization task, in which participants continued tapping after the end of the sequence, following which they reported whether they had noticed a change. These findings fit nicely the distinction between the conscious conceptual content of a HOT and the non-conceptual content of an unconscious first-order mental state. According to the definition above, we can say that C (the perceptually registered but unnoticed change) refers to the non-conceptual part of the content of M, which was not a part of one of Y's HOTs and thus was not experienced. Hence, again, the idea that the content of HOTs is conceptual remains intact.[24]

It is worth deviating for a moment to point out that there is support for the view that even the qualitative aspects of the perceptual states (unconscious) are conceptually captured.[25] As Alva Noë correctly notices, "concepts are brought into play even when you fail to notice, when you see, as it were, automatically or 'without thought'" (1999: 10). As he points out, the fact that one does not stumble over the letters of a text and that one is not forced to attend deliberately to each and every one of them is constitutive of being a comfortable reader. Furthermore, the "cocktail-party effect", where one suddenly becomes conscious of hearing one's name, suggests that conceptualization and its mechanisms can occur unconsciously. Equally suggestive is the case of the piano tuner (discussed in Chapter 4). Although the tuner may not be aware of the fact that the piano is out of tune because he is not really listening to it, if the piano stopped playing he would notice it. As Dennett says, he would even be able to tell you exactly which notes were out of tune. Such examples suggest not only that sensory states can occur unconsciously, but also that there are cases where their qualitative aspects are captured by our conceptual capacities. One must have been hearing articulated words and not mere sounds or nothing at all in order to be able to become conscious of hearing one's name and the tuner's ability can be explained by appealing to her training and to the learning of new concepts. Had the tuner not been through all this training and concept learning, she would not be able to tell which notes were out of tune. As Martin Heidegger remarks:

> We never really first perceive a throng of sensations, e.g., tones and noises, in the appearance of things ...; rather, we hear the storm whistling in the chimney, we hear the three-motored aeroplane, we hear the Mercedes in immediate distinction from the Adler. Much closer to us than all sensations are the things themselves. We hear the door shut in the house and never hear acoustical sensations or even mere sounds. (1964: 656)

Yet it might be objected that it is still not clear whether our conceptual capacities can indeed capture all the fine detail and richness of the content of our perceptual experiences. The non-conceptualist motivation here may be that even if there is a distinction between conscious and unconscious perceptual content, our perceptual experience still appears to be more fine-grained than our conceptual repertoire: it seems implausible that we have a distinct concept for every shade of colour we experience in our visual field, for example. It naturally follows that not all content of perceptual experience is conceptual. Therefore, the content of one's experience transcends one's conceptual capacities, the non-conceptualist may argue. Evans writes in this famous passage:

> The proposal is implausible, because it is not the case that we simply find ourselves with a yen to apply some concept ... Nothing could more falsify the facts of the situation ... Do we really understand the proposal that we have as many concepts as there are shades of colour that we can sensibly discriminate? (1982: 229)[26]

Similarly, Alex Byrne writes:

> Can the content of a visual experience – for instance my visual experience as I gaze on a sunny day towards the San Gabriel mountains – be captured in a single thought? ... [T]he concepts that I can deploy may be inadequate to characterise fully the content presented by the visual sensuous manifold, just as one may lack the resources to describe exhaustively the content of a painting. And certainly if my thoughts are all expressible in *English*, that would seem to be right. Call this the *inexpressibility problem.*
>
> (1997: 116–17)

Of course, our language lacks the conceptual repertoire to describe in detail what we consciously see. But, similarly, it lacks the repertoire to specify in detail what we believe that we see when we go beyond simple examples such as seeing that there is a red patch. However, when necessary we may augment our repertoire by temporally adding a concept of how things look by *ostension*. Suppose I have a tree in my back garden. Suppose that I have gazed at that tree almost every day for years; I do not, however, know what kind of tree it is. But, owing to the fact that I see that tree almost every day, I can exercise the capacity to think of that tree and this, further, gives me the ability to cross-contextually identify the species of that tree. Now, suppose that one day a friend sees the tree and, to my question, replies "That's a sycamore." I then become aware of the tree's name. Does this mean that it is only now that the species of the tree in question has been conceptualized? No. According to our initial definition, a concept is a Fregean sense (mode) of presentation and a thinker possesses it if it is a constituent of the intentional contents of judgements and beliefs of the thinker. And evidently in this case, I can have beliefs and other attitudes whose contents contain THAT TREE[27] as a constituent.

It is certainly true that, linguistically, perceptual experience is inexpressible as feelings are (apparently) so. But possession of a concept does not require possession of a *linguistic expression*: to have a concept of something (e.g. of a shade of colour) and therefore to have *that* something available in memory or for it to enter the contents of judgements and beliefs, it need not have a name or a linguistic expression. It is worth noting an instance coming from cognitive psychology. Benjamin Whorf (1956) suggested that the linguistic system is not merely a reproducing instrument for ideas but, rather, is itself the shaper of ideas, the programme and guide for the individual's mental activity. Whereas there is much more to be said on the connection between language and thought, I shall refer here only to cases where present-day stone-age tribes (e.g. the Dani of Irian Jaya, a stone-age Melanesian people), having a very limited capacity of linguistic expressions and more particularly an impoverished vocabulary respecting shades of colour – for example the Dani construe all shades of colour under DARK and BRIGHT –

proved to have the same (or almost the same) capacity of discriminating and recognizing shades of colour as modern English speakers have, thus showing that language does not have a major influence on how shades of colour are perceived (e.g. Davidoff *et al.* 1999).

Dretske (1995) and Peacocke (1992, 2001) further object that that there is plenty of empirical evidence to suggest that in order to master an observational concept (e.g. SCARLET) one must be able to see instances of this concept, and the ability to perceive those instances does not require that one has *already mastered* or possessed the observational concept. One can perceive an instance of scarlet without possessing the concept SCARLET. In this connection, it is worth quoting Noë:

> [T]he experience you have when you are aware of the observational property but do not possess the observational concept, is not (and cannot) be the experience *as of* that property. The experience must be as of something, however (owing to the intentionality of perceptual experience). What dependency commits us to is the requirement that you have the conceptual resources – however primitive – to appreciate how things are experienced as being. (1999: 264)[28]

What it is like for one to have a particular sensation of red may say nothing about the particular shade. A sensation can be conscious as a sensation of scarlet but not of a particular fine-grained shade scarlet12, say, or it may be conscious as a sensation of red but of no particular shade. Further, as we have seen, when necessary we may augment our repertoire by temporally adding a concept of how things look by ostension. Following McDowell (1994), we can say that the fineness of grain of the content of perceptual experience can be captured conceptually by the use of perceptual demonstrative concepts such as THAT SHADE. As McDowell puts it:

> In throes of an experience of the kind that putatively transcends one's conceptual powers – an experience that *ex hypothesi* affords a suitable sample – one can give a linguistic expression to a concept that is exactly as fine-grained as the experience, by uttering a phrase like "that shade", in which the demonstrative exploits the presence of the sample ... (1994: 56–7)

> A capacity to embrace a shade within one's thinking (as *that* shade, we may say in favourable circumstances) is initiating by the figuring of an instance of a shade in one's experience ... the capacity to have that particular shade in mind is a standing one, which requires

> no more than possession of the concept of a shade together with
> the subjects standing powers of discrimination. Experience raises
> this standing potential to a degree of actuality.   (*Ibid.*: 59)

Plausibly, any degree of subtlety in one's current perceptual experience could
be capture by a demonstrative concept, such as THAT SHADE or COLOURED
THUS.

There is an alleged problem for the conceptualist here; namely, that col-
our-indiscriminability is not transitive. The problem is this: for colour sam-
ples x, y and z the normal observer may find y indiscriminable from x and z
and yet x discriminable from z. Now, according to the conceptualist thesis,
two things fall under the same perceptual demonstrative concept just in case
they are indiscriminable. This, however, leads to a contradiction since x and
y fall under the same concept, z falls under the same concept as y and yet x
does not fall under the same concept as z. And since the conceptualist thesis
seems not to be able to accommodate the claim that colour indiscriminabil-
ity is not transitive, any colour could fall under the perceptual demonstrative concept (one could link the colour of a thing with that of the perceived
sample through a chain of things that are indiscriminable from one another).
As Jérôme Dokic and Elisabeth Pacherie (2001) emphatically observe, in this
case, everything would have the same colour. In effect, we have a sorites
paradox. The conceptualist reply here is that something that counts as having
a shade does not thereby count as a *sample* of the shade, bringing into the
shade's extension anything indiscriminable from it. The original shade that
falls under the demonstrative colour concept Cx, even if it is indiscriminable
from the sample colour that falls under concept Cy, will not do as a *sample*
of the original shade. Grasp of the demonstrative concept "that shade" is
provided by the experience of perceiving the colour sample, and under the
same demonstrative concept falls anything that is indistinguishable from *that*
sample *at the time of perceiving it*. Thus construed, the contradiction disappears (see McDowell 1994: esp. 170–71).

According to some philosophers, however, the fine-grained content of
perceptual experience cannot be captured in terms of such demonstrative
concepts because concepts, necessarily, correspond with entirely context-
independent classifications of things (e.g. Dokic & Pacherie 2001; Kriegel
2004). The main non-conceptualist idea here is that our so-called demonstrative concepts fail to meet certain criteria for concepthood, most importantly
the requirement for re-identification or cross-contextual classification of
things, and hence they cannot really qualify as concepts. Since concepthood
seems to require cross-contextual classification of things, it would appear
that demonstrative concepts have context-dependent norms of application,
and thus they cannot meet this requirement. Therefore, they cannot qualify

for concepthood. There have been several conceptualist attempts in the recent literature to meet this requirement (e.g. McDowell 1994; Brewer 1999). While much more needs to be said on how we are to construe this requirement, and surely much depends on how we are to construe it, there are two general points I would like to make.

First, the challenge is to show that a demonstrably defined concept (of a shape) can have indefinitely many applications in different contexts in one's experience. What is it to demonstrate the concept of a particular *shape*? I think we do it by demonstrating a *sample object* with that shape: the shape of that$_1$. More fully, in "the shape of that$_1$" the phrase "that$_1$" is a Kaplanesque demonstrative[29] of an *object*, not of a concept. But the definite description "the shape of that$_1$" refers to the wanted CONCEPT: the concept of the shape of the object in question. (Compare, "the president of France", where "France" refers to a country, but the whole description refers to something else, Nicolas Sarkozy.) So "the shape of that$_2$", where "that$_2$" refers to a different object, and therefore has a different sense from "the shape of that$_1$", may nonetheless pick out the same shape concept, that is, have the same referent, as "the shape of that$_1$". These definite descriptions express higher-order concepts, not the shape concept in question, which is their referent, not their senses. So we have not yet shown that the shape concept in question has been added to our conceptual repertoire. We have not yet used it in a judgement, but only referred to it. But having referred to it, we can now introduce the shape concept in question into our conceptual repertoire like this: for all objects x, x has SHAPE$_1$ if and only if the shape of x = the shape of that$_1$. Now we have enlarged our conceptual repertoire. We can employ the new concept in judgements of shape: e.g. THAT$_3$ (another object) has SHAPE$_1$.[30]

Second, it might be objected that although some demonstrative concepts are in this sense concepts proper, it is hard to see how such demonstrative concepts as THAT SHADE (or COLOURED THUS), THAT SOUND (or SOUNDS THUS) or THAT TASTE (or TASTES THUS) can be employed in cross-contextual classifications of things. On the face of it, it seems plausible to say that the content of one's experience may include, for instance, the shade scarlet13 without one's being able to cross-contextually identify or classify that shade. In other words, it seems reasonable to suggest that one would be unable to tell whether one is encountering the same colour if one were to be shown tomorrow the same, or a very similar sample of scarlet. Thus the idea seems to be that whereas one can discriminate scarlet13, one cannot recognize or re-identify that shade: one's discriminatory capacities outstrip one's conceptual repertoire (similar considerations apply to the demonstratives THAT TASTE and THAT SOUND).

But why should we think that our visual perceptual *experience* includes scarlet13 any more than our tasting-some-wine *experience* includes the fine qualitative properties that wine tasters experience? It is simply untrue that the experienced wine taster and I experience the same qualitative properties when tasting a wine and it is simply untrue that the piano tuner and I experience the same qualitative properties when we listen to the piano. It is plain that learning more about music theory enables us to hear chords differently and with more richness and the same considerations hold regarding wine tasting or appreciating a work of art: the richer our conceptual repertoire, the more fine-grained the differences among the qualities of our sensory states. Depending on the level of conceptual sophistication, two subjects can experience a painting for instance, in greater and lesser detail. Salvador Dali's visual experience of looking at one of his extraordinary paintings is much more refined than mine. Dali presumably has the ability to discriminate and re-identify scarlet13, whereas I may not have the ability to even experience scarlet13.[31] All in all, this objection seems to show only that grasp of the concepts fades with time. It seems to raise a memory problem, not a concept-hood problem. Cross-contextual classification seems not to be necessary for concepthood in that a person may not remember exactly or may not retain the capacity to recognize things as having that shade, and so on. Indeed, the very idea that we have a drawer out of which to drag concepts in order to re-identify things sounds counter-intuitive.

Looking out over the Grand Canyon at sunset, I consciously see that it looks *just so*, and believe that I see it looking *just so*. Although a temporary addition to my conceptual repertoire, this is the exercise of a genuine concept by Evans's tests (1981); for the short while I have it I can apply it to other particulars, as when I remember that yesterday Central Park did not look just so or, as the light changes, when I judge that the canyon now no longer looks so. We should not be fooled by my expressing the concept as "looking just so" into exaggerating the specificity of the ostensive concept. As my eyes saccade around the scene, there may be many changes in how it looks that I do not register. Dennett (1991a) reports being the subject in an experiment in which his head was held fixed while he looked at a page of text displayed on a computer screen. A camera tracked his eye movements and a program was able to note the trajectory of his saccades and accurately predict where on the computer screen he would next look. While his eyes were in transit the word displayed at the "landing" site was changed. It seemed to him that the text on the page was unchanging: things looked just so and continued to look just so. To any other observer the page was flickering as words changed here or there four or five times a second. Illusions, too, can be used to define temporary ostensive concepts.

Finally, there is empirical evidence (Raffman 1995) that suggests that we are aware of a far more fine-grained difference among qualitative properties when they occur together (when we characterize things comparatively) than when they occur one at a time. This fits our considerations well. According to most philosophers (e.g. Campbell 1997; Dokic & Pacherie 2001), propositional content is content with a subject–predicate structure. As Dokic and Pacherie emphatically observe, the demonstrative "this is thus" has conceptual or propositional content. Bearing in mind the intimate relation between our conceptual repertoire and what kind of qualitative properties we can experience, it appears that the main reason that we can have more fine-grained experiences when we characterize things comparatively is that we employ our conceptual capacities to characterize shades of colour, for instance, comparatively: for example, this shade of red is *lighter* or *brighter* than that (recall the case of the Dani tribe). Since "this is thus" and "that is *F*" are conceptual, "this is lighter or brighter than that" is conceptual too. Therefore, it does seem that our conceptual capacities are sufficient to make us aware of all the fine-grained variations of the qualitative properties that we experience.

NOTES

1. This is assuming that Charles Darwin's story about the evolution of the species is for the most part true. Recently, some neurologists have suggested that an adult *Homo habilis* might, in principle, be able to understand such truths. I remain neutral. If you find yourself agreeing with them, replace "ancestor *Homo habilis*" with "human babies".

1. THE NATURE OF THE MIND

1. What counts as a reason for doubting? The notion of "doubt" that Descartes seems to have had in mind was, roughly, that if it is conceivable that some future experience could show that what we claim as knowledge could be false, then our claim cannot be to entire certainty, and therefore we do not have knowledge.
2. Another version of this argument might be this: I know that minds exist without knowing that bodies exist, therefore I can exist even if bodies do not. This argument should be rejected for the same reason. Some philosophers attribute to Descartes a number of other not very powerful arguments: for instance, that since a body is spatially divisible, and a mind is spatially indivisible, then mind could exist even if the body did not; or that since I can doubt that I have a body, but I cannot doubt that I exist, then I can exist even if bodies do not exist. It is easy to find what is wrong with these arguments; none of them is valid.
3. Note the distinction between *qualitative* and *numerical* identity: X and Y are *qualitatively* identical to the degree that they share their properties. They might be exactly similar, particularly regarding their perceptible properties; for example, identical twins are qualitatively identical to a high degree and so are two new MP3 players – they share their colour, shape, size, weight and so on. X and Y are *numerically* identical if they are one and the same thing (MP3 player, chair, person). Identical twins are *not* numerically identical. Everything is numerically identical to exactly one thing: itself. When you ask "Is X *numerically identical* to Y", you are thereby asking "Is X and Y one and the same thing?" Obviously, if there is something true of X that is not true of Y and/or vice versa, then X and Y cannot be one and the same thing.
4. We might speculate that the conflict between religion and science, after the Renaissance, contributed to the creation of the traditional categories of mental and physical

and to the two kinds of reality: mental and material. The territory of the mental (or of the soul) was thought to belong to religion, or at any rate, not to science. Ancient Greek philosophers for instance, were dualists, but in a different sense. The dualism of Anaxagoras, for instance, was a dualism of mind and matter but mind, like matter, was thought to be corporeal; their difference was a matter of degree (depending on fineness and purity) not of kind.

5. Some philosophers are only property dualists. On this view, there is only one kind of substance in this world, physical substance, but there are essentially two different kinds of *properties* inhering in it, mental and physical properties. As a result, for a property dualist, the mind cannot survive the death of the body, not being a different substance (against Descartes). This view is a species of monism – the view that all things in the world are substances of one kind, typically physical or material – and has recently gained popularity owing mainly to its alleged ability to better handle mental causation problems. See §1.5 for discussion.

6. It does seem that direct causal interaction between mind and body is a better candidate to explain such facts than say, Leibnizian pre-established harmony between mind and body, that is, the idea that there is no causal interaction between them and that God has pre-established a harmony between the mind and the body, which are rather like two clocks that were synchronized by the shopkeeper in the morning. And it is certainly a much better candidate than Malebranche's occasionalism, according to which there is no direct causal relation between minds and bodies, and when a mental event, say your will to raise your arm, occurs, that only serves as an occasion for God to intervene and cause your arm to rise.

Notably, Descartes thought that the causal interaction between mind and body takes place in the pineal gland, a small reddish-grey gland (about the size of a pea) located near the centre of the brain. The pineal gland was known in the ancient times as the "third eye" and was thought to have mystical powers. We now know that in some animals the pineal gland contains magnetic material and is a centre for navigation.

7. This is very rarely performed, and is normally a last resort in very serious cases of epilepsy. However, damage to the corpus callosum can result in *alien hand syndromes* (see pp. 22–3 for discussion).

8. There naturally follows his remark, "When a patient like this eventually dies, will one hemisphere end up in hell and the other in heaven?"

9. There are cases where it seems that ordinary people can experience the effects of a split consciousness. Michael Lockwood (1989) describes a man, who once hypnotized, was asked to place his right hand in a bucket of icy water for a considerable period of time. When asked if he felt any discomfort he verbally denied it, but when asked to write down how he felt he immediately complained of pain and asked to remove his hand.

10. One should then look for independent reasons in support of P1. Searle's Chinese room argument might do the trick (see §1.4). Regarding P2, it might be objected that even if one shows that minds are divisible, there is still a property that only material objects have; namely, extension in space. But the same considerations seem to apply: one must already assume that the human being is not a mere material thing. It seems that one is presupposing the distinction between mind and body rather than arguing for it. Dualists generally object that it just does not make sense to attribute properties such as size, shape and weight to minds; to do so is to commit what Gilbert Ryle (1949) called a "category mistake".

11. Of course, as things stand there is a difference between identities such as "Water = H_2O" and identities between mental states and particular brain states, for instance "pain = C-fibre firing", in that, for one thing, we do not think that water *correlates* with H_2O; they are one and the same thing, whereas contemporary neuroscience is

teaching us that the feeling of pain *correlates* with C-fibre firing. The first case implies that there is only one thing there (water or H_2O), and the second that there are two things (pain and C-fibre firing). Hence, it might be argued, it is conceivable that the feeling of pain can exist without C-fibre firing existing. As we shall see in the next section, some physicalists suggest that such *correlations* hold because, in fact, they are *identities*. If that is right, then P1 loses its intuitive appeal.

12. Simply put, according to the theory of relativity, faster than light *mere noise* is no threat to causality, but faster than light *signals* are deeply paradoxical.

13. Notably, Descartes seems to have denied the possibility of the philosophical zombie (1998: esp. 32). The zombie hypothesis has been central in discussions on consciousness, especially in the past twenty years, and it is immediately related to the explanatory gap problem. I shall be discussing it more clearly throughout the book. There are, however, other arguments related to the zombie argument, which I shall be touching on in this chapter, such as Jackson's *knowledge argument* and Kripke's *modal argument* (see §1.3).

14. The target of the Wittgensteinian attack was, of course, Russellian sense data, which, like Cartesian minds or souls, are essentially private mental objects, not open to third-person inspection and investigation.

15. *Transcranial magnetic stimulation* is a non-invasive method like fMRI to excite neurons in the brain, whereby electric currents are induced in the tissue by quickly changing magnetic fields. A large number of studies have now shown that similar methods could be used to treat motor deficits and various neurological conditions, such as migraine, stroke and Parkinson's disease. See Wassermann *et al.* (2008) for discussion.

16. There are other kinds of overdetermination but they all face similar problems. *Pre-emptive* overdetermination, for instance, employs the idea that the mental cause is in fact a *would be* cause, hence dropping the "both occur" requirement. For instance, in the example of the firing squad above, where two bullets enter the same organ, one enters a fraction of a moment earlier than the other effectively causing the death. The other follows and it is causally relevant in the sense that it *would* cause the death or causally contribute, but it arrived too late. In this case, however, it is obvious that there is no *causing* left to do.

17. Notably, contemporary epiphenomenalist William Robinson (2004b) thinks that direct causation of utterances by events is not always required in order for those events to be known. He writes, "we accept claims to knowledge if we think the chain of events leading up to the utterance of the claim is of a kind that would not occur if the claim were not true" (*ibid.*: 166). True. But this counterfactual dependence can hardly be said to be sufficient for knowledge. The same report would be made independently of whether a pain was occurring in that a zombie-twin would produce the same report. Later, in Chapter 6, I shall be arguing that what *constitutes consciously seeing* a red patch, for instance, is for one to believe that one is seeing the red patch on the rational ground of being visually aware of the red patch.

18. This very inability to explain how something spatial can give rise to something non-spatial has led some philosophers to suggest that the problem of the relation between physical and mental properties is beyond our powers of understanding. See §5.5 for discussion.

19. Behaviourists drew heavily on Ivan Pavlov, whose work had shown that you could condition dogs to salivate not just at the sight of food but at the sound of a bell that preceded food. Watson, for instance, argued that all human behaviour is built on just such conditioning.

20. According to the verification theory of meaning, a statement is *meaningful* if and only if it is *empirically verifiable* (or analytic, i.e. true by definition, e.g. "red roses are

red", or "1 + 1 = 2'). A statement is empirically verifiable if we know what observations would lead us, under certain conditions, to accept it as being true, or reject it as being false. This means that all metaphysical statements, for instance, statements about Cartesian minds or God, are meaningless, because no observations can lead us to accept or reject these statements (even in principle). We do not know under which conditions these are true or false, therefore, the argument goes, these statements are strictly speaking nonsense. So every meaningful psychological statement has to be empirically verifiable, and, as such, it should be defined solely in terms of behavioural statements, that is, those referring to behavioural phenomena (observable physical phenomena). Thus, "pain talk" has to be translated into "behaviour talk"; for example "He is in pain" should be replaced with sentences such as "He is crying out in agony".

21. Notice that on this view, we seem to have better access to the mental states of others than we do to our own. This has a false ring to it in that we typically know more about our own mental states than we do about the mental states of others.

22. Note the difference between *reductionism* and *eliminativism*. Reductionism is a theory that *explains* a phenomenon whereas eliminativism *explains it away*: whereas, according to reductionism, mental states are best regarded as talking about their corresponding brain states, eliminativism has it that mental states are best regarded as talking about nothing that actually exists – mental states are a product of bad theorizing. Eliminativism is anti-reductionist because it holds that there is no way that psychological theories can be reduced to neural or physical theories, or at any rate there is no point in doing so. An eliminativist about X denies the existence of X whereas a reductivist about X does not deny the existence of X, but tells us something about X that we did not previously know.

23. Notice, first, that this is a case of reduction, not of elimination: we learned something about Hesperus (i.e. that it is Phosphorus); we did not deny the existence of Hesperus. Second, in Frege's example, under both modes of presentation knowledge is public, whereas in the pain–C-fibre firing example, under one mode (pain) knowledge is private, and under the other (C-fibre firing) it is public.

24. Another way to put this is to say that mentality *supervenes* on the physical goings on in our brains. For further discussion see §1.5.

25. The fact that mental phenomena *correlate* with physical goings on in one's brain is consistent with dualist theories in the philosophy of mind, such as epiphenomenalism (and substance dualism, provided we do not hold on to the mental-to-physical dependency relation). It might be, for instance, that the correlation holds because C-fibre firing *causes* pain. Consider, smoking (A) *correlates* with lung cancer (B) and a heavy night's drinking (A) correlates with a hangover (B). In both cases, we normally say that A causes B and in both cases A and B are not one and the same thing. The point is this. The fact that A correlates and depends on B does not necessarily imply that A and B are one and the same thing.

26. Recall, for instance, the case of *transcranial magnetic stimulation* (from §1.1), where excitation of neurons in the brain induced by electrical currents brings about certain movements, such as arm or finger movements. In these cases, even more interestingly, the patients initially reported that they were feeling "urges", say, an urge to move the left arm, an urge to move the index finger and so on, and when the researchers increased the current a little in each case, this is exactly what happened: the urge turned into action, the very action the patients had reported they wanted to perform.

27. I discuss this point at length in §1.5.

28. With hours of practice, however, they may come to know *how* to shoot the ball, but in this case, they will acquire a new ability, not learn a new fact.

29. Note that a few years after the formulation of his argument, Jackson himself argued

that we should be suspicious of giving "intuitions about possibilities [like the Mary case] too big a place in determining what the world is like" (1998: 43–4). A similar line or response, about which I shall have more to say in the coming chapters, is that Mary's predicament of learning a new fact is purely *epistemic* and that her epistemic advance on leaving the room does not reflect any grasp of an unknown ontological feature of the world. This is one of the main positions on the explanatory gap problem: the fact that we cannot currently explain conscious experience in physical terms does not have any ontological implications.

30. The same point can be raised against behaviourism in that the thesis requires that we associate a *unique* behavioural pattern with every distinct mental phenomenon and it is plain that pain behaviour for instance, can be vastly different among species.

31. Self-consciousness is closely related with the concept of "personhood" that distinguishes us from non-human animals. It requires the ability that enables us to attribute mental states in everyday life and to reflect on our mental lives and the mental lives of others, that is, a "theory of mind".

32. Here is the argument formalized:
(Let $Q(x)$ be the subjective/qualitative character of x, what it is like to undergo x.)

P1. $\forall x,y \, [Q(x) \neq Q(y) \rightarrow x \, y]$

P2. $\forall x,y,w,z \, [x$ is human & y is animal & x undergoes w & y undergoes z $\rightarrow Q(w) \neq Q(z)]$.

Conclusion. $\forall x,y,w,z \, [x$ is human & y is animal & x undergoes w & y undergoes z $\rightarrow w \neq z]$.

33. This might seem too quick, but the underlying idea is simple. I defend the thesis that human conscious experience is conceptually structured in Chapter 6. There, I provide necessary and sufficient conditions for human conscious experience.

34. Notice that the functionalist is not so much concerned with *what there is* as with *what characterizes* a certain type of mental state. So although most functionalists, like Lewis, are physicalists, in that it does seem that some sort of matter is required to play the causal role, functionalism is not incompatible with dualism.

35. You cannot fail to notice the dualist intuitions that underline this response. It seems that there is some sort of an *emergent subjective aspect* to the brain that cannot be fully captured in pure functional terms. Still, it is hard to see why the right sort of functional organization of the constituents of any artificial system cannot give rise to that aspect. As we shall see more fully in Chapter 5, it is hard to make sense of Searle's account. He is not a brain-identity theorist and he is not a substance dualist. All in all, it might be fair to construe Searle's view as a species of property dualism (see §1.5).

36. We saw previously that it is conceivable that certain patterns of behaviour are there but the mental states are not (e.g. cases of actors and robots). We have further seen that it is conceivable that one's C-fibres are firing but one is not in pain (e.g. Kripke's argument). Now we see that it is conceivable that a state can play its causal role without there being anything that it is like for one to be in that state. Hence, it is conceivable that one is in a state that is behaviourally, physically and functionally identical to a conscious state without there being anything it is like for one to be in it. Voila! The philosophical zombie.

37. Notably, for Searle, but not for Kim, the supervenience relation is just *causation*. But then Searle cannot be a property dualist without violating the principle of the causal closure of the physical in that arguably, according to the principle, no causal chain can ever cross the boundary between the physical and the non-physical.

38. This principle states that no single event can have more than one sufficient cause occurring at any given time unless it is a case of causal overdetermination. But, arguably, causal overdetermination is not an option. The exclusion principle does not

favour the mental or the physical cause but the principle of the causal closure of the physical excludes the mental cause, enabling the physical cause to prevail.

39. Note that Kim thinks that (only) the fundamental level of microphysics is causally closed and we need this in order to have the required causal premise available.

2. PHENOMENAL CONSCIOUSNESS: THE HARD PROBLEM

1. This refers to sensory modality-based imaginations or mental representations; thinking of or imagining the taste or the redness, for instance, is a mental qualitative state.

2. More precisely, Dennett rejects the idea that qualia are essentially conscious, that is, that if one is in a state with qualia then one is in a conscious state. He does not think that, say, perceptual experiences and bodily sensations *per se* do not exist. I shall address Dennett's claim in Chapter 3

3. For one thing, there are many creatures that can detect changes in the environment while awake to which we would hesitate to ascribe the property of being conscious. There are certainly borderline cases, but the cases of insects, bees and caterpillars are suggestive enough. The point is that "creature" consciousness *can* be applied to creatures whose mental states are in some respect like the non-conscious states we are in when we are awake. It is then plain that the puzzling aspect of consciousness does not lie in creature consciousness.

4. For a detailed discussion of the kind of explanation required see Chapter 5.

5. In a similar spirit, Chalmers has suggested that what it means for a state to be phenomenal is for it to feel a certain way. In general, says Chalmers, a phenomenal feature of mind is characterized by what it is like for a subject to have that feature (1996: 12).

6. Block writes: "P-conscious properties are distinct from any cognitive, intentional, or functional property" (1995: 230). For Block, "P-consciousness, as such, is not consciousness of" (*ibid.*: 232). In a later version of this paper (2002), Block repeats both claims. P-conscious properties are then not representational in that they are not about things (e.g. properties of external objects). P-conscious properties are *intrinsic* properties of the state, they are not properties represented by the state or by the content of the state.

7. We are leaving aside the problem of how A-consciousness can interact with P-consciousness since the first is *dispositional* and the second is *occurrent*. As Anthony Atkinson and Martin Davies (1995) point out, this makes the relation between P-consciousness and A-consciousness the relation between the ground of a disposition and the disposition itself.

8. In Chapter 4, after I have introduced representationalism, it will become apparent that Block's claim that P-consciousness can occur without A-consciousness is far from convincing. There are, however, more serious problems with Block's notion of P-consciousness and I shall now turn to these.

9. It is worth noting that this is the current trend in contemporary philosophy of mind. Joseph Levine, for instance, takes qualitative character to contain subjectivity, namely "the phenomenon of there being something it's like for me to see the red diskette case. Qualitative character concerns the 'what' it's like for me: reddish or greenish, painful or pleasurable … Being an experience, its being reddish is … a way it's like for me" (2001: 7). I take Block's and Chalmers's views as exemplary, however, partly because they have a very similar conception of "experience" in spite of having entirely different views about what these qualitative properties or qualia are: Block is a brain-identity theorist and Chalmers is a property-dualist.

10. Block may have in mind more imaginative experiences, such as *hearing* number words spoken or *visual imagery* of the numerals.

11. Recall that according to Block, for instance, qualitative properties can be "a series of mental images or sub vocalizations". For example, someone may suddenly realize that she has left her favourite red-coloured T-shirt at the gym. There is then plausibly something it is like for her to have this realization and it may be said that there is a qualitative property involved, namely redness. If this realization then involves some-how *imagining* the redness, then this would amount to a sensory-modality-based mode of imagination. But clearly this experience of realizing does not reduce to the qualitative content of what is thus imagined.

12. Generally, as we shall see more fully in Chapter 5, conceivability suggests a need for an explanation, which is typically called for whenever it is conceivable that things could have gone the other way. And if one asserts that the hard problem of consciousness just is the problem of mental qualitative properties one must at the very least bridge, if not close, this explanatory gap.

3. PHENOMENAL CONSCIOUSNESS AND THE "SUFFICIENCY" CLAIM

1. This is relatively uncontroversial. Almost all philosophers agree on this point.

2. See for instance the "burning house" experiment (Marshall & Halligan 1988). Also, Berti & Rizzolatti (1992).

3. In fact, the suggestion quite forcefully put is that this is evidence that we can recognize the emotions of others without needing to be visually aware of them. For an excellent review of recent empirical evidence that non-consciously perceived emotional stimuli induce distinct neurophysiological changes and influence behaviour see Tamietto & de Gelder (2010).

4. There are now a large number of findings suggesting that unconscious representations of changes affect performance (Beck *et al.* 2001; Fernandez-Duque *et al.* 2003).

5. Visuomotor transformation is the network in the brain where visual information is converted into motor commands of arm and hand movement towards objects.

6. It appears that visual awareness is not a property of specific processing systems; its occurrence presupposes that the ventral stream, for instance, is capable of interacting with the various processing streams. For a proposal of how the parietal lobe (which is part of the dorsal stream of our visual system) contributes to visual awareness see Kanwischer (2001).

7. Notably, numerous findings suggest that brain imaging (fMRI scans) can currently reveal, to a certain extent, how one's choices are influenced by one's subconscious processes (emotions, instincts, desires, etc.). See, for instance, Phelps *et al.* (2000). It is expected that brain scans will be able to reveal on an individual basis what really makes people behave in a certain way despite the fact that, in some cases, their cognitive system tells them otherwise (e.g. cases of confabulation and self-deception).

8. Block has also appealed to cases of general anaesthesia (1995) and aerodontalgia. Aerodontalgia refers to cases of dental patients who reported experiencing toothaches years after their dental operations owing to sudden changes in atmospheric pressure, for example, in high-altitude flying. These patients underwent general but not local anaesthesia. The locations of the pain reported correspond to the sites where dental operations were carried out. Block suggests that these patients actually experienced pain (their pains were P-conscious) during the operation, but they were not A-conscious because of anaesthesia. He writes: "they found recreation of pain of previous dental work only for dental work done under general anesthesia, not for local anesthesia, whether or not the local was used alone or together with general anesthesia. Of course, there may have been no pain at all under general anesthesia,

only memories of the sort that would have been laid down if there had been pain. But if you hate pain, and if both general and local anesthesia make medical sense, would [you] take the chance on general anesthesia? At any rate, the tantalizing suggestion is that this is a case of P-consciousness without A-consciousness" (1995: 242).

9. Similar considerations apply if we regard *S* and *S** as a single mental state. In this case, the subject is aware of being in a state with such and such qualities, which do not include any qualities that correspond with the second object: the object the subject reports not seeing.

10. "For oneness" or "for the subject" is built into the full Nagelian formula, that is, the Nagelian what-it-is-likeness implies that there is something it is like *for one* to undergo the mental state. And Block seems to agree with Nagel in several places. In discussing whether a swampman (a molecular duplicate of a typical human made of swamp) can have phenomenally conscious states, for instance, Block states explicitly that the point at issue is whether or not "there is something it is like *for Swampchild* when 'words' go through his mind or come out of his mouth" (1998: 665, emphasis added). In an another paper, with reference to Wilder Penfield's (in Penfield & Erickson 1941) case of the epileptic driver who, despite having a seizure while driving, managed to arrive home safely, Block writes, "suppose he gets home by turning right at a red wall. Isn't there something *it is like for him* to see the red wall – and isn't it different from what *it is like for him* to see a green wall? ... no reason at all is given to think that their P-conscious states lack vivacity or intensity" (1995: 240, emphasis added). However, Block's later conception of consciousness seems to leave out the subjective aspect of our experiences.

11. It is also worth noting that Block makes clear at the beginning of his paper that the question he is going to consider is this: "since [Fodorian] representations are *cognitively inaccessible* and therefore *utterly unreportable*, how could we know whether they are conscious or not?" (2007: 481, emphasis added). "Cognitively inaccessible and utterly unreportable representations", then, may still be conscious according to Block. Block is not alone in this. For example, Fred Dretske's conception of (phenomenal) consciousness is very similar to Block's. Dretske too holds that one need not be aware of a first-order mental qualitative state in order for it to be an experience. Dretske says, for instance, that "what we are asking, remember, is not merely whether perception of something can occur without awareness of it, but whether conscious perception can occur alongside a belief that one is aware of nothing" (2006: 159). I discuss Dretske in Chapter 4.

12. Nagel's formula characterizes Block's higher-order conceptions of consciousness, that is, what he calls reflexivity or monitoring consciousness (which involves representation of one's mental states).

13. It might be objected that in the same sense there is no logical room for the idea of an unconscious mental state. I would be happy to endorse Block's line of thought to the effect that mental qualitative properties (and not experiences) can occur unconsciously. In the next three sections, I shall provide more reasons for this idea.

14. There is a third-person aspect of the "mind", according to Chalmers, but the properties that deal with this aspect are either nothing over and above brain states or cognitive properties that are specifiable in terms of their causal roles. Chalmers thinks that subjectivity cannot be explained from a third-person perspective; phenomenal properties are not amenable to a scientific explanation. Block disagrees with this idea but his account leaves subjectivity out.

15. Chalmers acknowledges that sense-data properties and qualia have many characteristics in common and disagrees with the approach that rejects the idea that qualia are private and essentially or intrinsically conscious: "I tend to believe in the qualia

Dennett wants to quine. I don't necessarily buy all four properties straight up (it depends on how you analyze them), but I have some sympathy for privacy, immediate apprehensibility, and intrinsicness; ineffability is tricky. I don't think Dennett has good arguments against the first three (in the relevant sense)" (informal communication, http://users.sfo.com/~mcmf/cqmail3.html [accessed November 2010]).

16. Note that the idea that mental qualitative properties cannot occur unconsciously is shared by Searle (1992, 2006), Levine (2001), Robinson (2004b), Kim (2005) and others.

17. The experiments cited earlier exhibiting similar effects suggest that the effects of "seeing red" could occur in the absence of consciousness of red.

18. Note that some philosophers have argued against the *conceivability* of zombies (e.g. Dennett 1991a; Clark 2000). See also §5.3 and §5.4.

19. An instrumental interpretation of an explanation or theory withholds ontological commitment to the explanatory entities seemingly postulated by the theory or explanation, in contrast to a realist interpretation, which takes such posits at face value. If the question at issue is the real possibility of the existence of zombies, then the supporting explanation of the zombie scenario needs to be interpreted realistically.

20. I do not think there is anything incoherent in the idea that a certain variety of philosophical zombies are conceivable. There can be many varieties. Some can have only first-order states. Some can have higher-order thoughts (HOTs). In Chapter 6, I shall argue that we cannot conceive of a creature that has a suitable HOT but is unconscious.

21. A man in Manchester made legal history in the UK after being acquitted of murdering his father because he was sleepwalking at the time (see Smith-Spark 2005).

22. Note that Robinson (like Chalmers) by "phenomenal qualities" means "mental qualitative" properties. He too thinks that they are essentially conscious and hence they cannot occur unconsciously.

23. Another criterion is simplicity. That is, even if we have a theory that has the same explanatory force as Chalmers's theory but is simpler or that avoids any unwanted implications, that is, avoiding Chalmers's notion of phenomenal or mental qualitative properties (or qualia) then by abduction (argument to the best explanation) we ought to adopt this theory.

24. By "synthesis", Kant roughly meant the act of putting different representations together. In other words, discrimination requires information and information requires organizing, which is provided by acts of synthesis.

25. Kant sometimes uses "intuitions" interchangeably with "appearances" and "impressions".

26. Notice the distinction between attention and introspection. Shifts of attention may be able to explain why we are conscious of some sensory states only some of the time but those states need not be introspectively conscious. A state is introspectively conscious only if the HOT by virtue of which we become conscious of something is itself conscious. Introspective consciousness involves attention to the second-order rather than the first-order state.

27. This also suggests that the higher-order state must be a thought and not an inner-sense or higher-order perception (HOP) (Lycan 1996). This is because, roughly, the higher-order sensing (or perceiving) must function analogously with first-order sensing (or perceiving). But the different families of qualitative properties are all specific to a single modality. Hence it is hard to see how the higher-order sensing can capture the cross-modal character of experiences such as those presented in the preceding paragraphs. A HOT, however, can have any content whatever, thus capturing such a cross-modal character. For a detail discussion of the inner-sense view see §6.2.

28. Another such case comes from David Simons & Christopher Chabris (1999). In the

task they used, observers looked at a film of two groups of players, a black-clad and a white-clad group, each playing with their own ball in the same small room. Their task was to try to track the number of times one group exchanges the ball. While the observer was doing this task a man dressed in a gorilla suit walked through the room. Although the man with the gorilla suit walked in full view, the subjects often failed to notice this utterly obvious event. It is then very tempting to suggest that although the subjects *saw* the gorilla suit man, *seeing him* was not part of the total *experiential state*. Plausibly, the findings cited earlier suggest that not all mental qualitative properties registered in our visual states are part of our total experiential state.

4. EXPERIENCE AND FIRST-ORDER REPRESENTATIONALISM

1. However, he denied the existence of unconscious mental phenomena (see Brentano 1973).
2. There are representational states that do not have similar correctness conditions. Wishing, for example, that p cannot be said to have truth conditions but arguably it is a representational state. Of course, the contents of such representational states still have correctness conditions but the attitude towards p cannot be said to be true or false.
3. Note that two contents or intentional objects may have different – Fregean – senses (modes of presentation) but the same reference; it depends on how what is re-presented is presented. For instance, to appeal to Frege's famous example, one person may think of the planet Venus as "The Morning Star" and another as "The Evening Star".
4. This notion of "relation" is certainly not the one that we normally use when we talk about relations between two (or more) existing things. Ordinary relations cannot hold between existent and nonexistent objects, but the mind can contemplate nonexistent objects and states of affairs. The directedness of the mind is that feature by virtue of which states of mind can have intentional objects or be about nonexistent things. According to representationalists, the nonexistent objects need not be immaterial substances (Russellian sense data for instance); they can be non-actual or nonexistent physical things or states of affairs.
5. Note that this is not the only variety of representationalism. In general, strong representationalists *identify* conscious qualitative character with the representational property representing a *certain content* in a *certain way*. There are different types of content in play as there are also different ways that content can be represented. The weak version has it that conscious qualitative character merely *supervenes* on the representational property.
6. Many philosophers have claimed that such a theory gives rise to an unacceptable "veil of perception" between the mind and the world. Most sense-data theorists are committed to the claim that sense data are mind dependent: objects whose existence depends on the existence of states of mind. These entities do not happily fit with a naturalistic world picture according to which the world is entirely physical in its nature, and everything there supervenes on the physical and is governed by physical law. Moreover, the postulation of private mental objects faces further problems, such as Wittgenstein's (1953) private-language argument.
7. Positing a nonexistent intentional object to solve the problem of locating qualia ontologically will certainly raise eyebrows. Lycan (1996), for instance, argues that intentional inexistents are best thought of as denizens of other possible worlds. They exist, just not here in the actual world. It appears, though, that this response does not help. Take, for example, the case of phantom pain in a missing limb. The painfulness of the phantom pain is actual, existing in the here and now. Likewise, when someone has a hallucination

190

of redness, there is a certain actually existing property that he is aware of, in virtue of which his experience has the qualitative character that it has. (Cases of illusion and hallucination pose serious problems to the representationalist *argument from transparency of experience*; see §4.3.) I shall not, however, develop this point any further nor shall I explore the range of the possible representationalist manoeuvres here.

8. Lycan writes, "The great difficulty about qualia was in locating them ontologically. (Of what, exactly, is the greenness inhering in Bertie's after-imaging experience a property?) *And that is what is accomplished by the specifically representationalist part of strong representationalism* ..., not by the functionalist part ... locating the greenness was the crucial work" (2006, emphasis added). The *functionalist* part accounts for "what-it-is-likeness", that is, for there being something it is like for one to be in states with such qualities. This might be a certain *dispositional role* of the first-order representational state (e.g. Dretske 1995; Tye 2000) or a higher-order state (perception) via the operations of a faculty of "inner sense" (Lycan 1996). But the fact that Lycan's account of experience is a higher-order account as opposed to Tye's first-order account is not important at this point. What matters is that, on both accounts, qualitative properties can be represented both consciously and unconsciously and a certain functional role (however construed) accounts for the fact that in some cases (conscious representations) we experience those properties, that is, there is something it is like to have them.

9. Elsewhere Tye writes, "the qualities of which we are aware are not qualities of experiences at all, but rather qualities that, if they are qualities of anything, are qualities of things in the world (as in the case of perceptual experiences) or of regions of our bodies (as in the case of bodily sensations)" (2007). According to Tye, "in the case of perceptual experiences, the items sensorily represented are external environmental states or features" (1995: 137).

10. Another is this. Tye writes, "twinges of pain represent mild, brief disturbances; aches represent disturbances inside the body, ones that have imprecise volumes, beginnings and ends ... these differences are paired with felt differences ... perhaps it might be objected that what it is like for the masochist is different to what it is like for me, even if we are subject to sensory representations of exactly the same sort of tissue damage ... my reply is that the felt quality of the *pain* is the same for both of us. I find the felt quality horrible and I act accordingly. He has a different reaction. Our reactions involve further feelings, however. I feel anxiety and concern. He does not" (1995: 135).

11. Traditionally, one of the main problems of perception is whether these properties are properties of physical objects or some sort of mental entities: sense data. See Robinson (1994) for an excellent discussion.

12. I shall leave out of the discussion Tye's stronger claim that "we attend to the external surfaces and qualities and thereby we are aware of something else, the 'feel' of our experience" (2000: 51–2). The point is that even if one accepts that the qualitative character of the experience is wholly representational, this does not explain by itself (or in effect) what it is like to undergo a certain state with a certain qualitative character (see §4.4). What is more, Tye claims that someone *is* aware of the fact that her mental state is representing certain qualities but she *is not* aware of the experiences themselves. But if she is aware that her mental state is representing such and such qualities or that she undergoes a mental state with such and such qualities, why not say that there is something in addition to the representational properties, namely *introspective awareness*? What explanation is given for the fact that in this case she is *consciously* undergoing a certain mental state (supposing that we accept that all its properties are representational)? In other words, the awareness of undergoing a certain mental state is left unexplained.

13. Fiona Macpherson (2003) proposes another counter-example based on Hewitt Crane and Thomas Piantanida's "filling in" experiment (Crane & Piantanida 1983), which suggests that we can have experiences of novel hues, such as reddish-green. This is a problem for phenomenal externalism because it appears that no plausible candidate can be found for the objective (externally constituted) physical colour property that experiences of reddish-green (or yellowish-blue for that matter) represent.

14. I have argued elsewhere (2009) that the other main representationalist arguments, if successful, establish no more than a *symmetrical supervenience relation* between represented content and qualitative character, and that a supervenience relation alone (albeit symmetrical) does not suffice for identity. In a word, from "no change in how we experience the world with no change in the world *and* no change in the world with no change in how we experience the world", it does not follow that what we experience, or what we are directly aware of, are properties of the external world.

15. Generally, a concept might be thought of as a *Fregean sense*, a way of thinking about something (mode of presentation). Tye seems to succumb to this view owing mainly to the *argument from the fineness of grain of perceptual experience*. I consider this argument in §6.8, where I also consider the question of whether conscious experience has a non-conceptual content, that is, whether all qualitative aspects of a conscious qualitative state are such that we have concepts of them.

16. For the view that for a state to be conscious is for it to be poised to have an impact on the organism's decision-making processes see Dretske (1993, 2006) and Kirk (1994). For Tye, the functional role is played by the content and not by the state that bears the content.

17. This further suggests that the existence of conscious qualitative character is not conditioned by the existence of environmental features but rather by the nature of conscious subjects. Although the qualitative features of our perceptual experiences may be determined *externally*, what-it-is-likeness or experience is determined *internally*, that is by the nature of the conscious subject.

18. Compare what a HOR theorist says on the same topic: "even bodily sensations such as pains can at times go wholly unnoticed, and so can exist without being conscious" (Rosenthal 1991: 17).

19. Computer-animated virtual "persons" equally have a learning capacity. The degree of success of communication between virtual and human persons depends for the most part on the degree of sophistication of the virtual person's learning programme.

20. More recently Peter Carruthers (2004) has explicitly argued that there can be *suffering* without *subjectivity*, without, that is, what-it-is-likeness. I fail to find any intelligibility in the idea that there may be nothing it is like for a creature to be in a particular state, yet the creature may suffer being in it.

21. To remind the reader, in the case of visual extinction, subjects presented with identical objects on both sides of their field of vision report seeing only one. Patients report that they do not see anything on one side of the visual field but if asked to guess what is there they guess with considerable accuracy.

22. Recall that Block describes the main function of an A-conscious state as being available for use in reasoning and rationally guiding speech and action. Notice that, on Tye's account, "P-consciousness" is characterized by the same function. Hence, if we allow that "P-consciousness" cannot occur without "A-consciousness" and that they are characterized by the same main function, then, as I have argued previously, it makes much more sense not to distinguish between P-conscious states and A-conscious states in terms of different *kinds* of consciousness involved, but in terms of the objects of the same consciousness.

23. In a similar spirit, Dretske defines "aware *of*" (as opposed to "aware *that*") as follows:

"S is aware of X = S perceives X, and information about X is available to S as a reason (justification) for doing what she wants (chooses, decides) to do" (2006: 174). Bearing in mind Block's notion of A-consciousness, namely that a state is A-conscious if it is "poised to be available in reasoning and for the rational control of speech and action", we can notice two things. First, Dretskean experiences require Block's access consciousness (they cannot occur without it), and second, in line with our considerations, Dretske says that "information about X *must be available to S as a justificatory reason*" (*ibid.*, emphasis added). According to Dretske, as it were, mere guesswork will not do. I turn to Dretskean experiences in a moment.

24. Notably, "notice" and "identify", on Dretske's account, are taken to mean epistemic perceptions or awareness *that* one sees something, as opposed to being aware *of* something (non-epistemic perception). Although non-epistemic perceptions occur unconsciously, they are nevertheless conscious. Someone is in a conscious state, says Dretske, but is not aware *that* he is in that state. In such cases, he is only aware *of* the things he sees, not *that* he sees them.

25. Disjunctivists distinguish sharply between genuine *perceptual experiences*, on the one hand, and *non-perceptual experiences* that may be mistaken for genuine perceptions, on the other. These two types of experience are of fundamentally different natures because only the former take as constituents actual, external aspects of a perceiver's environment. Hallucinatory experiences are non-perceptual in nature because of their failure to do so. Thus disjunctivists deny a common factor to perception and hallucination (see Martin 1997).

26. As the previously cited experimental data suggest, the absent-minded driver's skilful driving may simply be a matter of the driver's exercising her sensorimotor abilities. This point becomes more evident when we look at cases such as Penfield's epileptic driver. There are many cases of epileptics who have a seizure while walking, driving or playing the piano. The patients continue their activities in a routinized, mechanical way despite a lack of consciousness or awareness (see for discussion Searle 1992). These patients are described by Penfield as having a "total lack of consciousness".

27. Dretske writes, for instance, that "[w]hat makes [mental states] conscious is not S's awareness of them, but their role in making S conscious – typically (in the case of sense perception), of some external object" (1997: 6).

28. Carruthers thinks that in this way we can avoid the cognitive overload objection to *actualist* HOR theories, which require that the higher-order states must be an occurrent thought (HOT) or perception (HOP). The objection targets especially actualist HOT accounts: it appears implausible that HOTs have the power to fully represent the detail of our experiences. To do so, they would have to represent an enormous amount of information. This is because, according to the actualist accounts, one needs to have a distinct activated higher-order belief for each distinct aspect of one's experience. According to Carruthers, it is implausible that all this activity takes place every time one has a complex experience. Although this objection might be tackled more easily by a higher-order *perception* theory, the actualist HOT theorist might respond that dispositional states are themselves mental states and it is unclear whether a dispositional model is more efficient: whether that is, it handles better matters of cognitive economy (see Rosenthal 2004).

29. Following David Lewis (1980), it might be objected that defining dispositions are those limited to "normal" members of the species. People fitted with meddlers are not normal. But then, as Lewis himself worries, what is "normal"? Why should someone fitted with a meddler not be a normal member of some other comparison set, the meddlers?

30. Tye (1995, 2000), for example, claims that phenomenal character (equated with what-

it-is-likeness on his account) is *one and the same* as representational content that meets certain specifiable conditions. It appears, then, that for different contents one has different experiences.

31. Think of the binding problem: what scientists attempt to solve is how our perceptual experiences can represent the various environmental features we experience at any given time bound together in a single consistent, unified setting.

32. The object could have been in such a position that light from it affected the central part of Freddie's retina so that, perhaps, there was no perception at all.

33. This is why Dretske's distinction between epistemic and non-epistemic seeing is useful. It can be argued that Freddie was aware *of* the cufflink but not aware *that* he saw it. This is all good as long as the fact that Freddie was aware of the cufflink is not taken to mean that Freddie experiences the cufflink, as Dretske suggests.

34. What is it like for one to experience and not experience pain at a given time? Perhaps some dispositionalists might allow that individuals have multiple personalities without having any psychotic disorders. But this is a very high price to pay.

35. What was it like *for me* to *experience* the setting around me when I walked into the room? If we succumb to a Dretskean (dispositionalist) view of experience, then we face the intolerable dilemma: either at t_1 I found myself having contradictory experiences (since I was aware that *p* and aware of not-*p* and, according to Dretske, not only awareness *that*, but awareness *of* is also sufficient for experience) or alternatively only aware *that* confers what-it-is-likeness in the Nagelian sense (Dretskean awareness *of* leaves the Nagelian what-it-is-likeness out). Further, when one is presented with ambiguous stimuli such as the duck–rabbit figure (or the Necker Cube) there is no instance where there is something it is like *for one* to experience seeing both the duck and the rabbit. What it is like for one to see that figure depends on one's judgement to the effect *that* one is aware of the rabbit, or that one is aware of the duck figure.

36. Note that this feedback-guided, gain-adjusted tracking performed by any combination of brain states can bring about such HOTs.

5. EXPERIENCE AND THE EXPLANATORY GAP

1. I discuss the HOP view (Lycan 1996), which construes experience as a certain kind of higher-order qualitative property, in §6.2.

2. There is also evidence that the inferior parietal cortex is involved in our ability to distinguish between self-produced actions and actions produced by others (for discussion see Meltzoff & Decety 2003).

3. See Kim (2005: ch. 4) for a number of possibilities.

4. This is the kind of reductionism favoured by those philosophers who argue that experience cannot be reductively explained. Hence, I will then take issue with this kind of reductionism in order to meet their challenge.

5. It might be objected that we cannot get deductive implications from microphysics to biology as Chalmers and Jackson imply, or even get deductive links from physics to chemistry, except for very simple cases, such as the hydrogen atom and so on. I shall not, however, address such worries here. I shall attempt to show that we can give an explanation for experience along the same lines.

6. With the proviso that the antecedent is not a contradiction and the consequent is not a tautology.

7. *C* will be a logical consequence of *P* & *T* & *I* only if the logical forms involved, alone, are enough to guarantee that *C* is not false when *P* & *T* & *I* are true. "Tom is unmarried" is entailed by "Tom is a bachelor", but "Tom is unmarried" is not a logical con-

sequence of "Tom is a bachelor". If "deduce" means derive by the rules of logic, one cannot deduce "Tom is a bachelor" from "Tom is unmarried". Strictly, there may be unknown and unknowable logical truths: so that a conditional is a logical truth does not imply that it is an *a priori* conditional. And there may be *a priori* conditionals that are not logical truths. An example is this: "if Tom is a bachelor then Tom is unmarried" is an *a priori* truth but not a logical truth.

8. In a similar fashion, Levine writes, "suppose I want to explain why water boils, or freezes, at the temperatures it does. In order to get an explanation about these facts, we need a definition of 'boiling' and 'freezing' that brings these terms into the proprietary vocabularies of the theories appealed to in the explanation" (1993: 131).

9. It is clear from other writings that all this is to be included in *P* (see e.g. Chalmers 2009).

10. The same objection applies as above: the requirement is that $(P \& \neg Q)$ is conceivable by a Laplacian demon.

11. Note the difference between panprotopsychism and panpsychism. According to the latter, everything is conscious down to a subatomic level. On this view, there is something that it feels like to be an electron or a proton. On Chalmers's panprotopsychism, electrons or protons are proto-conscious: they do not possess consciousness. Proto-conscious properties collectively constitute consciousness in the right kind of system.

12. Chalmers follows Russell in holding that the laws of physics describe the structural interrelations that obtain in the material world, but do not specify which intrinsic properties actually stand in those structural relations. So laws of mass, momentum and so on describe *structural roles*, and the *intrinsic properties* that realize these roles may *differ* from possible world to possible world. It may be that in the actual world these roles are be realized by the properties of mass$_\alpha$, momentum$_\alpha$ and so on, but in another possible world obeying the same laws of nature the very same roles are realized by the different intrinsic properties: mass$_\beta$, momentum$_\beta$ and so on.

13. See Anthony Brueckner (2001) for an argument (against Chalmers's Cartesian intuition) to the effect that conceiving the truth of *p* is not sufficient to establish the possibility of *p*. My point here is that the possibility of *p* provides no explanation whatever, let alone that its explanatory burden when it comes to mental causation is a lot heavier.

14. "Noumenal" here is used in a Kantian sense, according to which a *noumenon* or *thing in itself* is an unknowable, indescribable reality that, in some way, lies "behind" observed phenomena. By "cognitive closure" is meant that the human mind has its limits and, in a Chomskian fashion, that matters of human puzzlement are either solvable problems or unsolvable mysteries. McGinn thinks that owing to our limitations of understanding, the operations of the human mind are incapable, in principle, of taking us to a proper appreciation of what experience is and how it works.

15. However, what he adds to this is merely that we are not aware when we have an experience of either the spatial location or of the dimensions of our experience. This is no objection to his view, according to Searle, because there is no reason that we should be so aware.

16. It is worth noting that in Searle's latest book he states that his "biological naturalism", as he calls the view, provides a "germ of a solution" or "a naturalistic solution" to the mind–body problem (2004: 113). The solution consists of a set of four theses, which in essence are as follows: conscious states are real phenomena irreducible to neurophysiological states; they are entirely *caused* by neurophysological states and can be causally reduced to them; they are realized in the brain and portions of the brain system are conscious; conscious states are causally efficacious.

17. Recall that the claim is that no matter how much information we are given about

experience in physical, functional or *cognitive* terms, it will not explain experience: no conceptual connection can be established between physical, functional or *cognitive* facts and facts about experience.

18. It is worth noting that Chalmers's non-reductive (as oppose to reductive) explanation appeals to proto-experiential or proto-conscious properties or facts. Although a proto-conscious fact looks simpler than a conscious fact, Chalmers rightly calls his explanatory strategy non-reductive, since the notion of "simpler entities" he has in mind means facts or properties that are not conscious and make no appeal to experience.

19. Why not reduce experience to, say, brain states instead of reductively explain it (see for instance, Block & Stalnaker [1999] for such a proposal)? Well, first, I would like to meet the Chalmers and Jackson neo-Cartesian challenge head-on. Second, as Kim (2005) has convincingly argued, the identification of experiences with neurophysiological properties cannot be supported empirically by inference to the best explanation. Kim's point is that the type-physicalist identities do not play genuine explanatory roles. Explanations work by drawing connections between a set of facts (the explanans) and a distinct fact or facts (the explanandum). But the identities, if true, assert that the identified facts are really one and the same. So, there is no movement here from one fact to another, something that surely must happen in a genuine explanatory argument. Third, as we saw in Chapter 1, such reductivist accounts are susceptible to a whole host of problems.

6. EXPERIENCE AND HIGHER-ORDER REPRESENTATIONALISM

1. Some philosophers, however, have argued that the HOP theory ultimately reduces to the HOT theory (Güzeldere 1995).

2. As stated above, this awareness is spelled out in terms of an occurrent HOT or HOP about the first-order state. The challenge is to show that none of the abilities that one must possess for a suitable higher-order state to occur essentially require consciousness.

3. What is more, since Carruthers places demands that HOTs themselves be conscious – in other words, the creature must have the ability to reflect on his or her mental state, that is, have a "theory of mind" – then any creature without this ability cannot have experiences (non-introspectively conscious states). This is problematic in that, for instance, consider autism. It is suggested that the core impairment in this condition stems from the failure to acquire such a "theory of mind" (Baron-Cohen 1995). So, if that is right, then autistic patients (and some healthy five-year-olds) cannot find themselves in (phenomenally) conscious states; that is, there is nothing it is like to be them (see the end of §6.3 for discussion).

4. Note that Armstrong's (1968) absent-minded driver was one of the main motivations behind HOR. Armstrong challenged the assumption that although some of our mental states such as thoughts, desires and beliefs can occur unconsciously, our perceptual or sensory states are essentially conscious; if one is in such a mental state then one is in a conscious state. He argued that when someone is driving very long distances in monotonous conditions he can come to at some point and realize that he has driven many miles without being conscious of the driving. He was not conscious of any of the route nor of any of the obstacles he adeptly managed to avoid, but must surely have been *seeing*; otherwise he would have crashed the car. Armstrong suggested that there can be unconscious *perceptual* states, which are precisely the states of which subjects are not introspectively aware.

5. Note that Tye (2002) says, for instance, that in creatures like humans, *introspective accessibility* is a necessary condition for experience: it is required for a state to be conscious that it be available to introspective awareness (a view also held by Carruthers [1996, 2000]). This is interesting given that Tye and Carruthers seem to think that their theories are quite distinct.

6. Note that this is consistent with the idea that mental qualitative properties are both intrinsic properties of perceptual states and externally constituted properties of objects in the environment. The point is that these properties (the so-called qualia), whatever they turn out to be, do not somehow carry consciousness within themselves; that is, these properties are not essentially conscious.

7. It is indeed most natural to regard consciousness as a relational property and not as an intrinsic property of the state: the organism is *conscious of* the state. It certainly sounds strange to say that the states themselves are conscious: following Nagel, we said that an organism X is conscious if and only if there is something it is like to *be* that organism, that is, if and only if there is something is like *for X*. So to say that, for instance, the pain itself is conscious is to say, in effect, that there is something it is like *for* it or that there is something it is like to *be* it!

8. Only mental states can become conscious in such a way. One cannot become conscious of the non-mental liver state for instance, in the same unmediated way. If one's doctor informs one to this effect then one's knowledge is mediate (via the speaker understanding what the doctor said) – for example, "I believe that my liver state is in poor condition" – whereas, in contrast, "I feel a pain in my liver", for instance, is a mental qualitative state because it is immediate. While this is true of the contrast between propositional attitudes and mental qualitative states in many cases, it seems it does not generalize to make a principled contrast between propositional attitudes and mental qualitative states. Propositional attitudes can be immediate. Innate beliefs presumably are immediate, programmed in by evolution and triggered by external stimuli, but not mentally mediate.

9. When one is in non-introspectively conscious states one is unmediately conscious of mental states as belonging to oneself, but the self is no more than a raw bearer of such states. One is not conscious of that self in any other way (as opposed to how one is conscious of oneself when one is introspectively conscious). For further remarks on the Kantian idea that self-reference does not require self-identification see Shoemaker (1968) and Brook (2001). See also Rosenthal (2004, 2006).

10. Since Gallup's early experiment, numerous other chimpanzees have passed the mirror test as well as other species of great apes, including the orang-utan and some gorillas (see Gallup & Suarez 1986; Patterson & Cohn 1994). Most recently, it has been demonstrated that even Asian elephants possess the ability for self-recognition (Plotnik *et al.* 2006).

11. It is worth noting that experimental findings have shown that activation associated with self-perspectivity was located in the right temporoparietal junction zone and the medial parietal lobe. The self-perspectivity associated activation is closely related to the body-image region in the right parietal lobe and makes it thus plausible that self-perspectivity involves the body axis as literal centre of the ego-centred experiential space (see Vogeley & Fink 2003).

12. This provides us with everyday "folk" psychology talk. We have the ability to ascribe beliefs, desires, intentions and other propositional attitudes to ourselves and others. It has been suggested that by the age of five, most children have discovered that they and others are fallible subjects of experience (Frith & Frith 1999). Experimental studies of normal and abnormal development suggest that the abilities to attribute mental states to self and to others are closely related. Thus inability to pass standard "theory of

mind" tests, which refer to others' false beliefs, may imply lack of self-consciousness. Individuals who persistently fail these tests may, in the extreme, be unable to reflect on their intentions or to anticipate their own actions (Frith & Happé 1999). Interestingly, autism is a disorder with a specific impairment in the neurocognitive mechanism underlying this ability. Baron-Cohen (1995) suggested that the core impairment in this condition stems from the failure to acquire such a "theory of mind", which, in effect, suggests lack of self-consciousness or of the ability to become introspectively conscious. But, of course, this is not to mean that autistic people lack a basic self-reference sense of self. On the contrary, these findings, put together, strongly suggest that there are what might be called degrees of self-consciousness and that there is a layer of self-awareness more basic than self-consciousness.

13. Why have (b) "John believes that he sees *or seems to see* a red patch", rather than just "John believes that he sees a red patch"? Because he might consciously see a red patch but, owing to collateral beliefs, not believe his eyes. For instance, John took mescaline yesterday and had certain hallucinations. Today, while walking, he comes across what appears to be a dog dressed in a Pierrot costume, complete with ruff and cap, sitting on a wall talking to a cat. Of course, he takes himself to be hallucinating again and believes only that he *seems* to see a dog dressed in a Pierrot costume, and so on. But unknown to him, he is not hallucinating. There really is such a dog and he is consciously seeing it. Of course, in normal circumstances, someone who consciously sees that *p* will believe that she sees that *p*. We normally believe the evidence of our eyes.

14. Notice that those who claim that God exists sometimes claim a direct warrant that is akin to a direct perceptual warrant: they might claim that their belief is warranted by God having "spoken" to them or "revealed" himself to them directly in some other quasi-perceptual manner.

15. Compare this hypothesis with McGinn's mysterianism or brute physical–mental causations, or Chalmers's panprotopsychism and epiphenomenalism.

16. Recall further that Chalmers's formulation of the zombie argument and the Chalmers and Jackson argument stated in Chapter 5 require that "$P \& \neg Q$" and "$(P \& T \& I) \rightarrow C$", respectively be conceivable by a hypothetical Laplacian demon, and not by us since we cannot formulate P, and nor could we grasp it were it presented to us. Hence, no non-question-begging warrant for this claim appears to exist.

17. See Gennaro (1996, 2005), Rosenthal (2000, 2006); see also Lycan (1996). But there is a quicker move available here. Goldman's predicament seems to involve a category mistake; namely that, strictly speaking, mental states themselves can become conscious. But mental states, on a par with physiological states and rocks, do not become conscious; it makes little sense to ascribe consciousness to mental states themselves. For a mental state to be conscious there must be something it is like *for* the mental state and most obviously there is not. On our view, and in agreement with Nagel, *subjects* are conscious of mental states or aware of being in them. To say that a mental state is conscious is to say that one is conscious of it.

18. This is another instance of the terminological chaos in the field: I wonder what "subjective" is doing in "subjective conscious experience". Are there non-subjective conscious experiences too? According to Nagel, "what it is like to be that organism" is called "the subjective character of experience". And as we have already seen, the *subjective aspect* is, according to both Nagel and Chalmers, precisely what needs explaining.

19. I acknowledge that this is not a full answer to the "*how*" question. It is, however, an intuitive answer that has explanatory power and addresses the "*how*" question head-on. To be sure, there are well-known problems with giving an account of self-reference, but reducing the hard problem of consciousness to the problem of self-reference is clearly progress. Future work in the field of consciousness studies should focus more

on the nature of self-reference, since at the very least, in this case, we are dealing with a cognitive ability and we know roughly in which direction to go in order to get the result.

20. Note that, according to most philosophers, if there is first-person reference it is guaranteed reference, at least in the sense that the subject always succeeds in referring to herself when she refers first-personally (see e.g. Anscombe 1981; O'Brien 2007). Additionally, the subject knows when the subject refers to herself. So (P1) if there is first-person reference then it is guaranteed reference. (P2) There is first-person reference. (C) Hence, first-person reference is guaranteed reference. It seems that the only way to reject this argument is to argue that P2 is false. But this seems very counter-intuitive and since the possibility of misrepresentation involves the idea that P2 is false we can reject this possibility by *reductio*: since one of the salient features of first-person reference is that it is guaranteed reference, and since consciousness consists in the ability for self-ascription, the possibility of misrepresentation is ruled out.

21. According to some philosophers (e.g. Stalnaker 1998), the contents of both belief and perception are non-conceptual. I shall ignore this complication and assume that beliefs, at least, are conceptual. A lot more needs to be said about what are the necessary and sufficient conditions for concepthood. According to most philosophers, for instance, availability in memory and cross-contextual classification are necessary, together with the requirement that X is a sense. See the discussion later in Chapter 6.

22. The terminological chaos that surrounds the term "perceptual experience" makes it hard to say what kind of content they have in mind. Peacocke's (1992) non-conceptualism, for instance, seems to refer to the non-conscious perceptual content I have in mind, whereas later Peacocke (2001) talks interchangeably about "perceptual content" and the "content of perceptual experience" as being non-conceptual.

23. In addition, David Marr's (1982) work on vision suggested that the visual content is insulated from other knowledge structures available to the person – that is, cognitively impenetrable – at various *early stages of visual processing*, for example those responsible for attending to, and tracking, objects in space and time. Marr's non-conceptual (cognitively impenetrable) content refers to a 21/2D unconscious representation of the world.

24. Almost three decades ago, before such findings were published, it appears that Gareth Evans's idea was that perceptual states with non-conceptual content are non-conscious until the subjects' conceptual capacities are brought to bear on them. It looks very much as if Evans's non-conceptual content (or informational content, as he called it) is not the content of conscious perceptual states as it is for most contemporary philosophers (recall my discussion of Tye's PANIC). This is most often overlooked as most contemporary philosophers (Martin 1992; Peacocke 2001) talk interchangeably about unconscious and conscious perceptual content and refer to it as the "content of perceptual experience".

25. Note that the evidence suggests the unconscious application of concepts to first-order mental states, not that the first-order perceptual states are themselves conceptual entities.

26. Notice that Evans (1982) asks whether we really understand the suggestion that we have as many concepts as there are shades of colour that we can *sensibly discriminate*. Evans talks about our discriminatory capacities, not our experiential capacities.

27. I follow here the convention of identifying concepts with small capital letters.

28. Relatedly, Peacocke (2001) complains that one can see the pyramid shape without possessing the concept PYRAMID. But this in no challenge to our considerations. There is an interesting analogy here. As in the case of the natural kind concepts (e.g.

water), our thinker may use a different concept from the *primitive* one in the formation of contents and propositional attitudes. Hence, our thinker can manage to satisfy
the possession condition of the "that" perceptual demonstrative by using other than
the primitive concepts. Our thinker may use a complex concept or one that deriva-
tively comes from other *primitive* concepts appealing to her conceptual resources.
For example, she may not manage to satisfy WATER, but she may manage to satisfy
THE LIQUID I LIKE TO DRINK BEST or THE PREDOMINANT CONSTITUENTS OF RIV-
ERS AND LAKES. Similarly, with respect to the concept PYRAMID (to use Peacocke's
example), one may manage to satisfy the possession condition of it by using THE
POLYHENDRON WITH ONE FACE – BASE – A POLYGON AND ALL THE OTHER FACES
TRIANGLES MEETING AT A COMMON VERTEX or THE SHAPE WITH THE TRIANGULAR
SIDES AND THE SQUARE BASE or even THE ANCIENT EGYPTIAN MONUMENTS' SHAPE.
In all these cases, one may not possess PYRAMID but one still, using complex concepts,
can satisfy the possession condition of something that has the same extension. Both
conceptual uses (primitive and complex concepts) have the same extension. Moreover,
the mental representation of, say, WATER and THE LIQUID I LIKE TO DRINK BEST, and
hence what enters the contents of judgements and beliefs, may be exactly the same.

29. For the demonstrative to present its demonstratum (that which is demonstrated), the
demonstratum must satisfy certain conditions. The mode of presentation picks out a
unique individual just in case the referent satisfies the reference-determining conditions of that mode of presentation. See David Kaplan's (1989) "demonstratives".

30. Note that according to the Fregean theory of demonstratives, in cases where a certain shape is perceived as "the shape of that$_1$" at t_1 and as "the shape of that$_2$" at t_2 (it
may be the shape of the same thing at different times [or from different perceptual
viewpoints at the same or different times] or the same shape of different things), the
identity statement involving those demonstratives is informative: that is, "the shape of
that$_1$ is the shape of that$_2$," is an informative statement. Since the statement is informative, its constituent demonstratives express a sense. Sean Kelly (2001) complains that
such perceptual demonstratives cannot take into account the full complexity of the
context and thus cannot account for the full phenomenology of perceptual experience. It appears, however, that they can incorporate the complexity of the context
at least, in the same sense and to the extent that HESPERUS (The Morning Star) and
PHOSPHORUS (The Evening Star) incorporate the complexity of the context.

31. It further appears that as we increase our conceptual repertoire we experience the
same qualitative properties *differently*. Consider two subjects A and B that possess the
concepts SHADE and RED and the concepts SHADE, RED and SCARLET, respectively.
We might as well say that A and B are in fact the same person at two different times:
an earlier time (t_1) when the person does not possess SCARLET and a later time (t_2)
when the person comes to possess SCARLET. According to Peacocke (1998), despite
the fact that B possesses the concept SCARLET and A does not, a scarlet object, for
example, is exactly the same for the two subjects. Peacocke says that independently
of the fact that A's repertoire stops at RED, what they both perceive is a single shade,
which they experience in the same way. This strikes me as implausible. For one thing,
B (e.g. a painter) can experience SCARLET in immediate distinction from, say, CRIM-
SON or MAROON, or part of B's experience could be that the ibis (a vivid scarlet bird)
looks like *this* shade of colour on B's painter's palette but not like *that*. For A there is
no such distinction to experience.

BIBLIOGRAPHY

Abbott, A. 2009. "Not Blind to Emotion". *Nature* online. www.nature.com/news/2009/090928/full/news.2009.956.html (accessed October 2010).

Anscombe, G. E. M. 1965. "The Intentionality of Sensation: A Grammatical Feature". In *Analytical Philosophy: Second Series*, R. J. Butler (ed.), 158–80. Oxford: Blackwell.

Anscombe, G. E. M. 1981. "The First Person". In her *Metaphysics and the Philosophy of Mind*, 21–36. Minneapolis, MN: University of Minnesota Press.

Armstrong, D. M. 1968. *A Materialist Theory of Mind*. London: Routledge & Kegan Paul.

Armstrong, D. M. 1981. "What is Consciousness?" In *The Nature of Mind*, D. Rosenthal (ed.), 55–67. Ithaca, NY: Cornell University Press.

Atkinson, A. & M. Davies 1995. "Consciousness without Conflation". *The Behavioral and Brain Sciences* **18**(2): 248–9.

Atkinson, R. 1993. *Introduction to Psychology*. Orlando, FL: Harcourt Brace.

Baars, B. 1997. "Contrastive Phenomenology: A Thoroughly Empirical Approach to Consciousness". In *The Nature of Consciousness*, N. Block, O. Flanagan & G. Güzeldere (eds), 187–202. Cambridge, MA: MIT Press.

Baron-Cohen, S. 1995. *Mindblindness: An Essay on Autism and Theory of Mind*. Cambridge, MA: MIT Press.

Barrett, L. F. 2006. "Are Emotions Natural Kinds?" *Perspectives on Psychological Science* **1**: 28–58.

Bayne, T. & D. Chalmers 2003. "What is the Unity of Consciousness?" In *The Unity of Consciousness: Binding, Integration, Dissociation*, A. Cleeremans (ed.), 23–58. New York: Oxford University Press.

Beck, D. M., G. Rees, C. D. Frith & N. Lavie 2001. "Neural Correlates of Change Detection and Change Blindness". *Nature Neuroscience* **4**: 645–50.

Berti, A. & G. Rizzolatti 1992. "Visual Processing without Awareness: Evidence from Unilateral Neglect". *Journal of Cognitive Neuroscience* **4**(4): 345–51.

Block, N. 1990. "Inverted Earth". In *Philosophical Perspectives 4*, J. Tomberlin (ed.), 53–79. Atascadero, CA: Ridgeview.

Block, N. 1994. "Consciousness". In *A Companion to the Philosophy of Mind*, S. Guttenplan (ed.), 210–19. Oxford: Blackwell.

Block, N. 1995. "On a Confusion About a Function of Consciousness". *Behavioral and Brain Sciences* **18**(2): 227–47.

Block, N. 1996. "Mental Paint and Mental Latex". In *Philosophical Issues 7: Perception*, E. Villanueva (ed.), 19–49. Atascadero, CA: Ridgeview.

Block, N. 1997. "Biology versus Computation in the Study of Consciousness". *The Behavioral and Brain Sciences* **20**(1): 159–66.

Block, N. 1998. "Is Experiencing just Representing?" *Philosophy and Phenomenological Research* **58**(3): 663–70.

Block, N. 2001. "Paradox and Cross Purposes in Recent Work on Consciousness". *Cognition* **79**(1–2): 197–219.

Block, N. 2002. "Concepts of Consciousness". In *Philosophy of Mind: Classical and Contemporary Readings*, D. Chalmers (ed.), 206–18. New York: Oxford University Press.

Block, N. 2003. "Mental Paint". In *Reflections and Replies: Essays on the Philosophy of Tyler Burge*, M. Hahn & B. Ramberg (eds), 165–200. Cambridge, MA: MIT Press.

Block, N. 2007. "Consciousness, Accessibility and the Mesh between Psychology and Neuroscience". *Behavioral and Brain Sciences* **30**: 481–99.

Block, N. & R. Stalnaker 1999. "Conceptual Analysis, Dualism, and the Explanatory Gap". *Philosophical Review* **108**(1): 1–46.

Brentano, F. 1973. *Psychology from an Empirical Standpoint*, A. C. Rancurello, D. B. Terrell & L. McAlister (trans.). London: Routledge.

Brewer, B. 1999. *Perception and Reason*. Oxford: Oxford University Press.

Brook, A. 2001. "Kant, Self-awareness, and Self-reference". In *Self-reference and Self-awareness*, A. Brook & R. DeVidi (eds), 9–30. Philadelphia, PA: John Benjamins.

Brueckner, A. 2001. "Chalmers' Conceivability Argument for Dualism". *Analysis* **61**(3): 187–93.

Byrne, A. 1997. "Some Like it HOT: Consciousness and Higher-Order Thoughts". *Philosophical Studies* **86**(2): 103–29.

Byrne, A. 2001. "Intentionalism Defended". *Philosophical Review* **110**(2): 199–239.

Byrne, A. 2004. "What Phenomenal Consciousness is Like". In *Higher-Order Theories of Consciousness: An Anthology*, R. Gennaro (ed.), 203–25. Philadelphia, PA: John Benjamins.

Campbell, J. 1997. "Sense, Reference and Selective Attention". *Proceedings of the Aristotelian Society*, supplementary vol.: 55–74.

Carruthers, P. 1996. *Language, Thought and Consciousness*. Cambridge: Cambridge University Press.

Carruthers, P. 2000. *Phenomenal Consciousness*. Cambridge: Cambridge University Press.

Carruthers, P. 2004. "Suffering without Subjectivity". *Philosophical Studies* **121**(2): 99–125

Carruthers, P. 2006. "Conscious Experience versus Conscious Thought". In *Consciousness and Self-Reference*, U. Kriegel & K. Williford (eds), 299–321. Cambridge, MA: MIT Press.

Chalmers, D. 1993. "Self-Ascription without Qualia: A Case-Study". *The Behavioral and Brain Sciences* **16**(1): 35–6.

Chalmers, D. 1995. "Facing up to the Problem of Consciousness". *Journal of Consciousness Studies* **2**(3): 200–19.

Chalmers, D. 1996. *The Conscious Mind: In Search of a Fundamental Theory*. Oxford: Oxford University Press.

Chalmers, D. 2002a. "Consciousness and its Place in Nature". In *Philosophy of Mind: Classical and Contemporary Readings*, D. Chalmers (ed.), 247–72. New York: Oxford University Press.

Chalmers, D. 2002b. "Developing a Science of Consciousness". Transcript, International Society for Complexity, Information, and Design. www.iscid.org/davidchalmers-chat.php (accessed October 2010).

Chalmers, D. 2004. "The Representational Character of Experience". In *The Future for Philosophy*, B. Leiter (ed.), 153–81. Oxford: Oxford University Press.

Chalmers, D. 2009. "The Two Dimensional Argument Against Materialism". In *The Oxford Handbook of the Philosophy of Mind*, B. McLaughlin, A. Beckerman & S. Walter (eds), 313–35. Oxford: Oxford University Press.

Chalmers, D. & F. Jackson 2001. "Conceptual Analysis and Reductive Explanation". *Philosophical Review* **110**(3): 315–61.

Churchland, Patricia 1983. "Consciousness: The Transmutation of a Concept". *Pacific Philosophical Quarterly* **64**: 80–95.

Churchland, Paul 2005. "Chimerical Colours: Some Novel Predictions from Cognitive Neuroscience". In *Cognition and the Brain: The Philosophy and Neuroscience Movement*, A. Brook & K. Akins (eds), 309–35. Cambridge: Cambridge University Press.

Clark, A. 2000. "A Case Where Access Implies Qualia?" *Analysis* **60**(265): 30–38.

Crane, T. 2006a. "Dualism, Monism, Physicalism". *Mind & Society* **1**(2): 73–85.

Crane, T. 2006b. "Is there a Perceptual Relation?" In *Perceptual Experience*, T. S. Gendler & J. Hawthorne (eds), 126–46. Oxford: Oxford University Press.

Crane, H. D. & T. P. Piantanida 1983. "On Seeing Reddish Green and Yellowish Blue". *Science* **221**: 1078–80.

Crick, F. & C. Koch 1990. "Towards a Neurobiological Theory of Consciousness". *Seminars in the Neurosciences* **2**: 263–75.

Dainton, B. 2004. "Higher-Order Consciousness and Phenomenal Space: Reply to Meehan". *Psyche* **10**(1). http://web.mac.com/barrydainton1/Research/Papers_files/Higher%20 Order%20Reply%20to%20Meehan.pdf (accessed October 2010).

Davidoff, J., I. Davies & D. Roberson 1999. "Colour Categories in a Stone-Age Tribe". *Nature* **398**: 203–4.

Davidson, D. 1970. "Mental Events". In *Experience and Theory*, L. Foster & J. Swanson (eds), 79–101. New York: Humanities Press.

Davidson, D. 1974. "On the Very Idea of a Conceptual Scheme". *Proceedings and Addresses of the American Philosophical Association* **47**: 5–20.

Dement, W. 1999. *The Promise of Sleep: A Pioneer in Sleep Medicine Explores the Vital Connection Between Health, Happiness and a Good Night's Sleep*. New York: Random House.

Dennett, D. 1987. *The Intentional Stance*. Cambridge, MA: MIT Press.

Dennett, D. 1991a. *Consciousness Explained*. New York: Little Brown.

Dennett, D. 1991b. "Lovely and Suspect Qualities". In *Consciousness*, E. Villanueva (ed.), 37–43. Atascedero, CA: Ridgeview.

Dennett, D. 1993. "The Message is: There is no Medium". *Philosophy & Phenomenological Research* **53**(4): 919–31.

Dennett, D. 1996. "Facing Backwards on the Problem of Consciousness". *Journal of Consciousness Studies* **3**(1): 4–6.

Dennett, D. 2001. *Kinds of Minds*. New Haven, CT: Phoenix Press.

Dennett, D. 2005. *Sweet Dreams: Philosophical Obstacles to a Science of Consciousness*. Cambridge, MA: MIT Press.

Descartes, R. 1996. *Meditations on First Philosophy*, J. Cottingham (trans.). Cambridge: Cambridge University Press.

Descartes, R. 1998. *Discourse on Method* and *Meditations on First Philosophy*, 4th edn. Indianapolis, IN: Hackett.

Dokic, J. & E. Pacherie 2001. "Shades and Concepts". *Analysis* **61**(3): 193–202.

Dretske, F. 1969. *Seeing and Knowing*. Chicago, IL: University of Chicago Press.

Dretske, F. 1993. "Conscious Experience". *Mind* **102**(406): 263–83.

Dretske, F. 1995. *Naturalizing the Mind*. Cambridge, MA: MIT Press.

Dretske, F. 1997. "What Good is Consciousness?" *Canadian Journal of Philosophy* **27**(1): 1–15.

Dretske, F. 2006. "Perception without Awareness". In *Perceptual Experience*, T. S. Gendler & J. Hawthorne (eds), 147–80. Oxford: Oxford University Press.

Dretske, F. *et al.* 1998. "An Interview with Fred Dretske". http://philosophy.stanford.edu/ apps/stanfordphilosophy/files/wysiwyg_images/dretske.pdf (accessed October 2010).

Elshof, G. T. 2005. *Introspection Vindicated: An Essay in Defense of the Perceptual Model of Self Knowledge*. Aldershot: Ashgate.

Evans, G. 1981. "Semantic Theory and Tacit Knowledge". In *Wittgenstein: To Follow a Rule*, S. Holtzman & C. Leich (eds), 118–37. London: Routledge.

Evans, G. 1982. *The Varieties of Reference*. Oxford: Oxford University Press.

Fang F. & S. He 2005. "Cortical Responses to Invisible Objects in the Human Dorsal and Ventral Pathways". *Nature Neuroscience* **8**(10): 1380–5.

Fernandez-Duque, D. & I. M. Thornton 2000. "Change Detection without Awareness: Do Explicit Reports Underestimate the Representation of Change in the Visual System". *Visual Cognition* **7**: 324–44.

Fernandez-Duque, D., G. Grossi, I. M. Thornton & H. J. Neville 2003. "Representation of Change: Separate Electrophysiological Markers of Attention, Awareness, and Implicit Processing". *Journal of Cognitive Neuroscience* **15**(4): 1–17.

Flanagan, O. 1992. *Consciousness Reconsidered*. Cambridge, MA: MIT Press.

Frege, G. 1892. "Uber Sinn und Bedeutung". *Zeitschrift für Philosophie und philosophische Kritik* **100**: 25–50.

Frith, C. D. & U. Frith 1999. "Interacting Minds – a Biological Basis". *Science* **286**(5445): 1692–5.

Frith, U. & F. Happé 1999. "Theory of Mind and Self-consciousness: What is it Like to be Autistic?" *Mind and Language* **14**(1): 82–9.

Gallup G. G., Jr 1970. "Chimpanzees: Self-recognition". *Science* **167**(3914): 86–7.

Gallup, G. G. Jr & S. D. Suarez 1986. "Self-awareness and the Emergence of Mind in Humans and Other Primates". *Psychological Perspectives on the Self 3*, A. G. Suls & J. Greenwald (eds), 3–26. Hillsdale, NJ: Erlbaum.

Gazzaniga, M. 1998. "The Split Brain Revisited". *Scientific American* **279**: 50–55.

Gennaro, R. 1996. *Consciousness and Self-consciousness*. Philadelphia, PA: John Benjamins.

Gennaro, R. 2005. "The HOT Theory of Consciousness: Between a Rock and a Hard Place?" *Journal of Consciousness Studies* **12**(2): 3–21.

Goldman, A. 1993. "Consciousness, Folk Psychology and Cognitive Science". *Consciousness and Cognition* **2**: 264–82.

Guttenplan, S. (ed.) 1994. *A Companion to the Philosophy of Mind*. Oxford: Blackwell.

Güzeldere, G. 1995. "Is Consciousness the Perception of what Passes in One's Own Mind?" In *Conscious Experience*, T. Metzinger (ed.), 335–57. Paderborn: Schöningh; Exeter: Imprint Academic.

Haagard, P., C. Newman & E. Magno 1999. "On the Perceived Time of Voluntary Actions". *British Journal of Psychology* **90**(2): 291–303.

Hardcastle, V. G. 1995. *Locating Consciousness*. Philadelphia, PA: John Benjamins.

Harman, G. 1990. "The Intrinsic Quality of Experience". *Philosophical Perspectives* **4**: 31–52.

Heck, R. G. 2000. "Nonconceptual Content and the Space of Reasons". *Philosophical Review* **109**(4): 483–523.

Heidegger, M. 1964. "The Origin of the Work of Art", A. Hofstadter (trans.). In *Philosophies of Art and Beauty*, A. Hofstadter & R. Kuhns (eds), 649–701. New York: Random House.

Hintikka, K. J. J. 1969. "On the Logic of Perception". In *Models for Modalities: Selected Essays*, K. J. J. Hintikka (ed.), 161–83. Dordrecht: Reidel.

Hollingworth, A. 2003. "Failures of Retrieval and Comparison Constrain Change Detection in Natural Scenes". *Journal of Experimental Psychology: Human Perception and Performance* **29**(2): 388–403.

Hollingworth, A. & J. M. Henderson 2002. "Accurate Visual Memory for Previously Attended Objects in Natural Scenes". *Journal of Experimental Psychology: Human Perception and Performance* **28**(1): 113–36.

Hohwy, J. & C. Frith 2004. "Can Neuroscience Explain Consciousness?" *Journal of Consciousness Studies* **11**(7–8): 180–98.

Humphrey, N. 2006. *Seeing Red: A Study in Consciousness.* Cambridge, MA: Harvard University Press.

Huxley, T. H. 1900. *Lessons in Elementary Physiology.* New York: Macmillan.

Jackson, F. 1977. *Perception: A Representative Theory.* Cambridge: Cambridge University Press.

Jackson, F. 1982. "Epiphenomenal Qualia". *Philosophical Quarterly* **32**: 127–36.

Jackson, F. 1998. *From Metaphysics to Ethics.* Oxford: Clarendon Press.

Jones, S. 1996. Interview with David Chalmers. *The Brain Project*, self-published CD-Rom.

Kant, I. 1929. *Critique of Pure Reason*, N. Kemp Smith (trans.). Basingstoke: Macmillan.

Kanwischer, N. 2001. "Neural Events and Perceptual Awareness". In *The Cognitive Neuroscience of Consciousness*, S. Dehaene & L. Naccache (eds), 89–114. Cambridge, MA: MIT Press.

Kaplan, D. 1989. *Themes from Kaplan.* Oxford: Oxford University Press.

Kelly, S. D. 2001. "The Non-conceptual Content of Perceptual Experience: Situation Dependence and Fineness of Grain". *Philosophy and Phenomenological Research* **62**(3): 601–8.

Kim, J. 1997. "Does the Problem of Mental Causation Generalize?" *Proceedings of the Aristotelian Society* **97**(3): 281–97.

Kim, J. 1998. *Mind in a Physical World.* Cambridge, MA: MIT Press.

Kim, J. 2005. *Physicalism, or Something Near Enough.* Princeton, NJ: Princeton University Press.

Kim, J. 2006. *Philosophy of Mind*, 2nd edn. Boulder, CO: Westview.

Kirk, R. E. 1994. *Raw Feeling: A Philosophical Account of the Essence of Consciousness.* Oxford: Oxford University Press.

Klinger, M. R. & A. G. Greenwald 1995. "Unconscious Priming of Association Judgments". *Journal of Experimental Psychology: Learning, Memory and Cognition* **21**: 569–81.

Kriegel, U. 2002. "PANIC Theory and the Prospects for a Representational Theory of Phenomenal Consciousness". *Philosophical Psychology* **15**(1): 55–64.

Kriegel, U. 2004. "Perceptual Experience, Conscious Content, and Non-conceptual Content". *Essays in Philosophy* **5**(1): 1–14.

Kripke, S. 1980. *Naming and Necessity.* Cambridge, MA: Harvard University Press.

Levine, J. 1993. "On Leaving Out What it's Like". In *Consciousness*, M. Davies & G. W. Humphreys (eds), 121–36. Oxford: Blackwell.

Levine, J. 2001. *Purple Haze: The Puzzle of Consciousness.* Oxford: Oxford University Press.

Lewis, D. 1972. "Psychophysical and Theoretical Identifications". *Australasian Journal of Philosophy* **50**: 249–58.

Lewis, D. 1980. "Mad Pain and Martian Pain". In *Readings in the Philosophy of Psychology*, vol. I, N. Block (ed.), 216–22. Cambridge, MA: Harvard University Press.

Lewis, D. 1986. "Causal Explanation". In *Collected Papers*, vol. 2, 214–40. Oxford: Oxford University Press.

Libet, B. 1985. "Unconscious Cerebral Initiative and the Role of Conscious Will in Voluntary Action". *Behavioral and Brain Sciences* **8**: 529–66.

Libet, B. 2001. "Conscious Intention and Brain Activity". *Journal of Consciousness Studies* **8**(11): 47–63.

Leibniz, G. 1965. *Monadology and Other Philosophical Essays*, P. Schrecker & A. M. Schrecker (eds & trans.). New York: Bobbs-Merrill Co.

Lipton, P. 1993. "Contrastive Explanation". In *Explanation*, D.-H. Ruben (ed.), 207–27. Oxford: Oxford University Press.

Locke, J. 1989. *An Essay Concerning Human Understanding*, P. H. Nidditch (ed.). Oxford: Clarendon Press.

Lockwood, M. 1989. *Mind, Brain and the Quantum: The Compound "I".* Oxford: Blackwell.

Lowe, E. J. 1995. "There are no Easy Problems of Consciousness". *Journal of Consciousness Studies* **2**(3): 266–71.

Lycan, W. G. 1996. *Consciousness and Experience*. Cambridge, MA: MIT Press.

Lycan, W. G. 1999. "A Response to Carruthers' 'Natural Theories of Consciousness'". *Psyche* **5**(11). http://theassc.org/files/assc/2434.pdf (accessed October 2010).

Lycan, W. G. 2001. "The Case for Phenomenal Externalism". *Noûs* **35**(1): 17–35.

Lycan, W. G. 2004. "The Superiority of HOP to HOT". In *Higher-order Theories of Consciousness*, R. Gennaro (ed.), 93–114. Amsterdam: John Benjamins.

Lycan, W. G. 2006. "Representational Theories of Consciousness". *Stanford Encyclopedia of Philosophy*. http://plato.stanford.edu/entries/consciousness-representational/ (accessed October 2010).

Macpherson, F. 2003. "Novel Colours and the Content of Experience". *Pacific Philosophical Quarterly* **84**(1): 43–66.

Mack, A. & I. Rock 1998. *Inattentional Blindness*. Cambridge, MA: MIT Press.

Marcel, A. 1983. "Conscious and Unconscious Perception: An Approach to the Relations Between Phenomenal Experience and Perceptual Processes". *Cognitive Psychology* **15**: 238–300.

Marr, D. 1982. *Vision: A Computational Investigation into the Human Representation and Processing of Visual Information*. New York: W. H. Freeman.

Marshall, J. & P. Halligan 1988. "Blindsight and Insight in Visuo-spatial Neglect". *Nature* **336** (29 December): 766–7.

Martin, M. G. F. 1992. "Perception, Concepts, and Memory". *The Philosophical Review* **101**(4): 745–61.

Martin, M. G. F. 1997. "The Reality of Appearances". In *Thought and Ontology*, M. Sainsbury (ed.), 81–106. Milan: Franco Angeli.

Meltzoff, A. N. & J. Decety 2003. "What Imitation Tells us About Social Cognition: A Rapprochement Between Developmental Psychology and Cognitive Neuroscience". *Philosophical Transactions of the Royal Society of London*. Series B, *Biological Sciences* **358**: 491–500.

McDowell, J. 1994. *Mind and World*. Cambridge, MA: Harvard University Press.

McGinn, C. 1989a. "Can We Solve the Mind-Body Problem?" *Mind* **98**(391): 349–66.

McGinn, C. 1989b. *Mental Content*. Oxford: Blackwell.

McGinn, C. 1991. *The Problem of Consciousness*. Oxford: Oxford University Press.

McGinn, C. 1995. "Consciousness and Space". *Journal of Consciousness Studies* **2**(3): 220–30.

McGinn, C. 2004. *Consciousness and its Objects*. Oxford: Oxford University Press.

Millikan, R. 1993. *White Queen Psychology and Other Essays for Alice*. Cambridge, MA: MIT Press.

Milner, A. D. & M. A. Goodale 1995. *The Visual Brain in Action*. Oxford: Oxford University Press.

Murphy, F. C., I. Nimmo-Smith & A. D. Lawrence 2003. "Functional Neuroanatomy of Emotion: A Meta-analysis". *Cognitive, Affective, and Behavioral Neuroscience* **3**: 207–33.

Nagel, T. 1974. "What is it Like to be a Bat?" *Philosophical Review* **83**(4): 435–50.

Nagel, T. 1986. *The View from Nowhere*. New York: Oxford University Press.

Nagel, T. 1987. *What Does it All Mean?* Oxford: Oxford University Press.

Neander, K. 1998. "The Division of Phenomenal Labor: A Problem for Representational Theories of Consciousness". *Philosophical Perspectives* **12**: 411–34.

Noë, A. 1999. "Thought and Experience". *American Philosophical Quarterly* **36**(3): 257–65.

Noordhof, P. 1999. "Micro-based Properties and the Supervenience Argument: A Response to Kim". *Proceedings of the Aristotelian Society* **99**(1): 115–18.

O'Brien, L. 2007. *Self-knowing Agents*. Oxford: Oxford University Press.

O'Regan, J. K. & A. Noë 2001. "A Sensorimotor Account of Vision and Visual Consciousness". *Behavioral and Brain Sciences* **24**(5): 883–917.

Pagin, K. G. 2009. "In Defence of a Doxastic Account of Experience". *Mind & Language* **24**(3): 297–373.

Patterson, F. G. P. & R. H. Cohn 1994. "Self-recognition and Self-awareness in Lowland Gorillas". In *Self-awareness in Animals and Humans*, S. T. Parker, R. W. Mitchell & M. L. Boccia (eds), 273–90. Cambridge: Cambridge University Press.

Peacocke, C. 1983. *Sense and Content*. Oxford: Oxford University Press.

Peacocke, C. 1992. *A Study of Concepts*. Cambridge, MA. MIT Press.

Peacocke, C. 1993. "Concepts". In *A Companion to Epistemology*, J. Dancy (ed.). 74–6. Oxford: Blackwell.

Peacocke, C. 1998. "Nonconceptual Content Defended". *Philosophy and Phenomenological Research* **58**(2): 381–8.

Peacocke, C. 2001. "Does Perception Have a Nonconceptual Content?" *Journal of Philosophy* **98**(5): 239–64.

Penfield, W. & T. C. Erickson 1941. *Epilepsy and Cerebral Localization*. Springfield, IL: Charles C. Thomas.

Perry, J. 1979. "The Problem of the Essential Indexical". *Noûs* **13**(1): 3–21.

Phan, K. L., T. D. Wager, S. F. Taylor & I. Liberzon 2002. "Functional Neuroanatomy of Emotion: A Meta-analysis of Emotion Activation Studies in PET and fMRI". *Neuroimage* **16**: 331–48.

Phelps, E. A., K. J. O'Connor, W. A. Cunningham *et al.* 2000. "Performance on Indirect Measures of Race Evaluation Predicts Amygdala Activity". *Journal of Cognitive Neuroscience* **12**: 729–38.

Platchias, D. 2009. "Representationalism, Symmetrical Supervenience and Identity". *Philosophia* **37**(1): 36–46.

Plotnik, J., F. B. M. Waal & D. Reiss 2006. "Self-Recognition in an Asian Elephant". *Proceedings of the National Academy of Sciences of the United States of America* **103**(45): 17053–7. www.pnas.org/cgi/reprint/0608062103v1 (accessed October 2010).

Putnam, H. 1963. "Brains and Behavior". *Analytical Philosophy*, Second Series, R. J. Butler (ed.), 211–35. Oxford: Blackwell.

Raffman, D. 1995. "On the Persistence of Phenomenology". In *Conscious Experience*, T. Metzinger (ed.), 293–308. Exeter: Imprint Academic.

Ramachandran, V. S. 2003. *The Emerging Mind*. London: BBC/Profile Books.

Repp, B. H. 2001. "Phase Correction, Phase Resetting, and Phase Shifts after Subliminal Timing Perturbations in Sensorimotor Synchronization". *Journal of Experimental Psychology: Human Perception and Performance* **27**(3): 600–621.

Rey, G. 1983. "A Reason for Doubting the Existence of Consciousness". In *Consciousness and Self-regulation: Advances in Research and Theory 3*, R. Davidson, G. Schwartz & D. Shapiro (eds), 1–39. New York: Plenum.

Robinson, H. 1994. *Perception*. London: Routledge.

Robinson, W. 2003. "Epiphenomenalism". In *Encyclopedia of Cognitive Science*, L. Nadel (ed.), 8–14. London: Nature Publishing.

Robinson, W. 2004a. "Colors, Arousal, Functionalism, and Individual Differences". *Psyche* **10**(2) (September 2004). www.theassc.org/files/assc/2598.pdf (accessed October 2010).

Robinson, W. 2004b. *Understanding Phenomenal Consciousness*. Cambridge: Cambridge University Press.

Rolls, E. T. 2005. *Emotion Explained*. Oxford: Oxford University Press.

Rosenthal, D. 1991. "The Independence of Consciousness and Sensory Quality". In *Consciousness: Philosophical Issues*, vol. 1, E. Villanueva (ed.), 15–36. Atascadero, CA: Ridgeview.

Rosenthal, D. 1997. "A Theory of Consciousness". In *The Nature of Consciousness*, N. Block, O. Flanagan, & G. Güzeldere (eds), 729–53. Cambridge, MA: MIT Press.

Rosenthal, D. 2000. "Metacognition and Higher-order Thoughts". *Consciousness and Cognition* **9**: 231–42.

Rosenthal, D. 2002a. "How Many Kinds of Consciousness?" *Consciousness and Cognition* **11**(4): 653–65.

Rosenthal, D. 2002b. "Explaining Consciousness". In *Philosophy of Mind: Classical and Contemporary Readings*, D. Chalmers (ed.), 406–21. New York: Oxford University Press. [Also published under the title "State Consciousness and What it's Like".]

Rosenthal, D. 2004. "Being Conscious of Ourselves". *Monist* **87**(2): 161–84.

Rosenthal, D. 2006. *Consciousness and Mind*. Oxford: Oxford University Press.

Russell, B. 1918. "The Philosophy of Logical Atomism". *Monist* **28**: 495–527.

Russell, B. 1998. *The Problems of Philosophy*. Oxford: Oxford University Press.

Ryle, G. 1949. *The Concept of Mind*. Chicago, IL: University of Chicago Press.

Salmon, N. 1989. "The Logic of What Might Have Been". *Philosophical Review* **98**(1): 3–34.

Schopenhauer, A. [1819] 1969. *The World as Will and Representation*, vol. 1, E. J. F. Payne (trans.). New York: Dover.

Seager, W. n.d. "On Dispositional HOT Theories of Consciousness". www.scar.utoronto. ca/~seager/carruthers.pdf (accessed October 2010).

Searle, J. 1980. "Minds, Brains and Programmes". *The Behavioral and Brain Sciences* **3**(3): 417–24.

Searle, J. 1983. *Intentionality*. Oxford: Oxford University Press.

Searle, J. 1992. *The Rediscovery of the Mind*. Cambridge, MA: MIT Press.

Searle, J. 2002. *Consciousness and Language*. Cambridge: Cambridge University Press.

Searle, J. 2004. *Mind: A Brief Introduction*. Oxford: Oxford University Press.

Searle, J. 2006. "Minding the Brain". *The New York Review of Books* **53**(17).

Sellars, W. 1956. "Empiricism and the Philosophy of Mind". In *Minnesota Studies in the Philosophy of Science, Volume I: The Foundations of Science and the Concepts of Psychology and Psychoanalysis*, H. Feigl & M. Scriven (eds), 253–329. Minneapolis, MN: University of Minnesota Press.

Sellars, W. 1963. *Science, Perception and Reality*. London: Routledge & Kegan Paul.

Shoemaker, S. 1968. "Self-reference and Self-awareness". *Journal of Philosophy* **65**: 555–67.

Shoemaker, S. 1994. "Self-knowledge and 'Inner Sense'". *Philosophy and Phenomenological Research* **54**(2): 249–314.

Simons, D. J. 2000. "Current Approaches to Change Blindness". *Visual Cognition* **7**(1–3): 1–15.

Simons, D. J. & C. F. Chabris 1999. "Gorillas in our Midst: Sustained Inattentional Blindness for Dynamic Events". *Perception* **28**(9): 1059–74.

Simons, D. J., C. F. Chabris, T. Schnur & D. T. Levin 2002. "Evidence for Preserved Representations in Change Blindness". *Consciousness and Cognition* **11**: 78–97.

Smart, J. J. 1959. "Sensations and Brain Processes". *The Philosophical Review* **68**(2): 141–56.

Smith-Spark, L. 2005. "How Sleepwalking Can Lead to Killing". BBC News, http://news.bbc. co.uk/1/hi/uk/4362081.stm (accessed October 2010).

Sperling, G. 1960. "The Information Available in Brief Visual Presentations". *Psychological Monographs: General and Applied* **74**(11): 1–30.

Stalnaker, R. 1998. "What Might Nonconceptual Content Be?" In *Concepts: Philosophical Issues*, vol. 9, E. Villanueva (ed.), 339–52. Atascadero, CA: Ridgeview.

Stoerig, P. 1996. "Varieties of Vision: From Blind Responses to Conscious Recognition". *Trends in Neuroscience* **19**: 401–6.

Stoerig, P. & A. Cowey 1989. "Wavelength Sensitivity in Blindsight". *Nature* **342**: 916–18.

Strawson, G. 1994. *Mental Reality*. Cambridge, MA: MIT Press.

Strawson, G. 2005. "Intentionality and Experience: Terminological Preliminaries". In *Phenomenology and Philosophy of Mind*, D. W. Smith & A. L. Thomasson (eds), 41–66. Oxford: Oxford University Press.

Strawson, P. F. 1974. *Freedom and Resentment and Other Essays*. London: Methuen.

Tamietto, M. & B. de Gelder 2010. "Neural Bases of the Non-conscious Perception of Emotional Signals". *Nature Neuroscience* **11**: 697–709.

Tamietto, M., L. Castelli, S. Vighetti *et al.* 2009. "Unseen Facial and Bodily Expressions Trigger Fast Emotional Reactions". *Proceedings of the National Academy of Sciences of the United States of America* **106**(42): 17661–6. www.pnas.org/content/106/42/17661 (accessed October 2010).

Tye, M. 1986. "The Subjectivity of Experience". *Mind* **95**: 1–17.

Tye, M. 1995. *Ten Problems of Consciousness*. Cambridge, MA: MIT Press.

Tye, M. 1998. "Précis of Ten Problems of Consciousness". *Philosophy and Phenomenological Research* **58**(3): 649–56.

Tye, M. 2000. *Consciousness, Color, and Content*. Cambridge, MA: MIT Press.

Tye, M. 2002. "On the Virtue of Being Poised – Reply to Seager". http://host.uniroma3.it/progetti/kant/field/tyesymp_replytoseager.htm (accessed October 2010).

Tye, M. 2003. "Phenomenal Character and Color – Reply to Maund". *Philosophical Studies* **113**(3): 281–5.

Tye, M. 2004. *Consciousness and Persons: Unity and Identity*. Cambridge, MA: MIT Press.

Tye, M. 2007. "Qualia". In *The Stanford Encyclopedia of Philosophy*, E. Zalta (ed.). http://plato.stanford.edu/entries/qualia/ (accessed October 2010).

Tye, M. 2009. "Representationalist Theories of Consciousness". In *The Oxford Handbook of Philosophy of Mind*, B. McLaughlin & A. Beckermann (eds), 253–67. Oxford: Oxford University Press.

Ungerleider, L. G. & M. Mishkin 1982. "Two Cortical Visual Systems". In *Analysis of Visual Behavior*, D. J. Ingle, M. A. Goodale & R. J. W. Mansfield (eds), 549–86. Cambridge, MA: MIT Press.

Vogeley, K. & G. R. Fink 2003. "Neural Correlates of the First-person Perspective". *Trends in Cognitive Sciences* **7**(1): 38–42.

Watson, J. 1913. "Psychology as the Behaviorist Views it". *Psychological Review* **20**: 158–77.

Wassermann, E. M., C. M. Epstein, U. Ziemann, V. Walsh, T. Paus & S. H. Lisanby 2008. *The Oxford Handbook of Transcranial Stimulation*. Oxford: Oxford University Press.

Wegner, D. M. 2002. *The Illusion of Conscious Will*. Cambridge, MA: MIT Press.

Weiskrantz, L. 1986. *Blindsight*. Oxford: Oxford University Press.

Weiskrantz, L. 1991. "Introduction: Dissociated Issues". In *The Neuropsychology of Consciousness*, A. D. Milner & M. D. Rugg (eds), 1–10. New York: Academic Press.

Whorf, B. L. 1956. *Language, Thought, and Reality*. Cambridge, MA: MIT Press.

Wittgenstein, L. 1953. *Philosophical Investigations*, G. E. M. Anscombe (trans.). Oxford: Blackwell.

INDEX